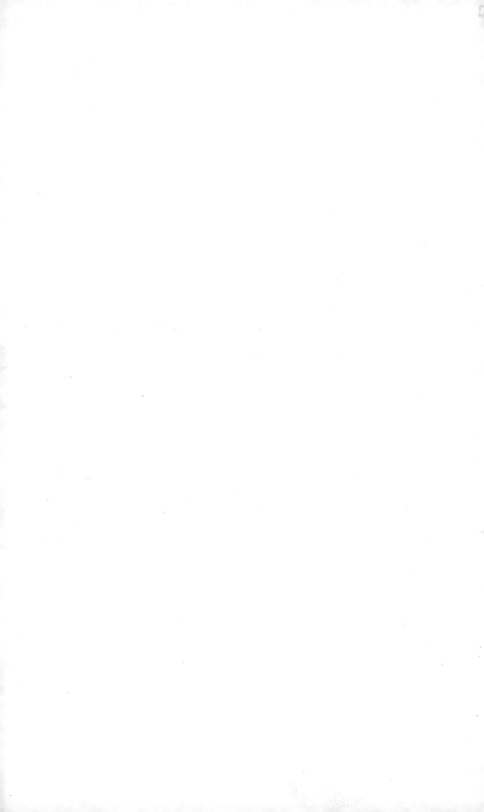

THE CONVERSATION

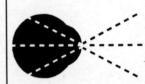

This Large Print Book carries the
Seal of Approval of N.A.V.H.

THE CONVERSATION

A REVOLUTIONARY PLAN FOR END-OF-LIFE CARE

ANGELO E. VOLANDES, M.D.

THORNDIKE PRESS
A part of Gale, Cengage Learning

GALE
CENGAGE Learning·

Farmington Hills, Mich • San Francisco • New York • Waterville, Maine
Meriden, Conn • Mason, Ohio • Chicago

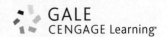

Copyright © 2015 by Angelo E. Volandes, M.D.
Thorndike Press, a part of Gale, Cengage Learning.

Thorndike Press® Large Print Mini-Collections.
The text of this Large Print edition is unabridged.
Other aspects of the book may vary from the original edition.
Set in 16 pt. Plantin.

LIBRARY OF CONGRESS CATALOGING-IN-PUBLICATION DATA

Names: Volandes, Angelo E., 1971– author.
Title: The conversation : a revolutionary plan for end-of-life care / by Angelo E. Volandes, M.D.
Description: Large print edition. | Waterville, Maine : Thorndike Press, a part of Gale, Cengage Learning, 2016. | Thorndike press large print mini-collection | Includes bibliographical references and index.
Identifiers: LCCN 2016032763| ISBN 9781410494788 (hardback) | ISBN 1410494780 (hardcover)
Subjects: LCSH: Palliative treatment. | Terminal care. | BISAC: SOCIAL SCIENCE / Death & Dying. | MEDICAL / Health Policy.
Classification: LCC R726.8 .V648 2016 | DDC 616.02/9—dc23
LC record available at https://lccn.loc.gov/2016032763

Published in 2016 by arrangement with Bloomsbury Publishing, Inc.

Printed in Mexico
1 2 3 4 5 6 7 20 19 18 17 16

32.99

To all my patients who allowed me to care for them during the darkest hour, in so much pain and suffering, and amid so much indignity wrought by disease and illness. Thank you for teaching me the heights and depths of human resilience.

Strive
in regards to disease
two things, to do good or not to do harm.
                    –Hippocrates, *Epidemics I*

CONTENTS

NOTE TO READERS

All the medical narratives in this book are grounded in actual events and real patients. I have altered the names, chronology, and identifying details of the patients — except my father — medical staff, and hospitals in order to maintain confidentiality. Wherever I use quotations from patients in the text, these are my recollections of discussions with patients from memory. I did not use any recording devices to document verbatim any patient discussions or comments presented throughout this book.

INTRODUCTION:
DEATH IN AMERICA

It was a blustery March morning at the crack of dawn, and my medical team was refueling with ample cups of coffee in the hospital cafeteria before reviewing our list of patients. Just as I took a scalding sip, the overhead speaker blared.

"Code Blue, Greenberg Five! Code Blue, Greenberg Five!"

Greenberg 5 was our floor in the hospital. We skipped the elevators — too slow — and ran up the stairway. Every second was critical. Although blue is the serene color of the Mediterranean Sea of my childhood summers back in Greece, in the hospital Code Blue has a more ominous meaning. It refers to a patient's blue face when blood — and the vital supply of oxygen it carries — has ceased to reach the heart and brain. Each second without oxygen is a second closer to death.

As the senior member of the team, my role

was to teach the medical residents how to be good doctors. Codes are a rite of passage for all physicians and, unfortunately, for many terminally ill patients. I suspected the code might be Lillian Badakian. She was a thirty-two-year-old mother of three with widely metastatic breast cancer. It had not responded to a radical mastectomy, radio-therapy, or numerous rounds of chemother-apy. In short, the skill and dedication of the nurses and doctors might get her through the Code Blue, but Lillian would almost certainly be dead within a few weeks, if not sooner.

We finally arrived on the floor and I at-tempted to catch my breath and compose myself. Now in my early forties, I was try-ing to keep pace with the medical residents on the team who were almost half my age. When we reached Lillian's room, her hus-band, Raffi, was pacing outside in the hall. As I entered I couldn't help but notice an old Christmas photo card pinned to the wall. Lillian, much healthier at the time, and Raffi had their arms around their three smiling sons. The whole family was fes-tooned in Santa hats. I pulled my gaze away from that proof of the family's happier times and focused on Lillian's heart monitor and the nurses gathered around her hospital bed.

The staff had already started CPR. One of the burly male nurses was leaning over Lillian performing chest compressions. "One, two, three . . ." he counted as sweat bloomed on his forehead. Another nurse was pumping air into Lillian's lungs with a green breathing bag. I told one of the younger doctors at the foot of the bed to take charge and run the code.

"Please continue chest compressions," the resident said, "and let's secure an airway. Get the heart monitor and pads ready in case we need to shock a V-fib arrest. Let's make sure we have two peripheral IVs and get the central line kit ready. Get me one of epi ready to go." She gave all the orders, exactly as she had been taught, and as I stood by her side, I remembered when I had been in her place. In time, she would be the senior doctor on the team and teaching other residents. This continual cycle of mentoring, as old as the practice of medicine itself, is its greatest tool.

I had only just met Lillian Badakian the previous day. In terrible pain and with virtually no statistical chance for survival beyond a few weeks or so, Lillian had reviewed her options for medical care and had chosen to press on with all available interventions in a bid to have one last Easter — now a seemingly interminable one month away — with her husband and children. In my heart of hearts, I knew then as we talked that there would be no Hollywood ending to Lillian's last wish. Now, even sooner than I had feared, I was a passive witness to her premature death from the same breast cancer that had already killed her mother, grandmother, and great-grandmother. Standing by her bed amid the orchestrated chaos of the Code Blue as Lillian began to slip away, I could not help but reflect on my own life's journey to this place.

Despite its focus on the twenty-first-century American approach to dying, the true subject of this book is life, because a life well lived deserves a good ending. When asked where and how they want to spend their last few months, nearly 80 percent of Americans respond that they want to be at home with family and friends, free from the institutional grip of hospitals and nursing homes, and in relative comfort. However, only 24 percent of Americans older than sixty-five die at home; 63 percent die in hospitals or nursing homes, sometimes tethered to machines, and often in pain. The reasons for this discrepancy between the type of medical care people want at the end of life and the type of medical care they actually receive are many, and include hospital culture, medical reimbursement schemes, and legal concerns; but the discrepancy is largely due to the failure of doctors to have discussions with patients about how to live life's final chapter. This is one of the most important problems facing American medicine today.

Despite the billions of dollars that are invested in new technologies in America's finest hospitals, the most important intervention in medicine today happens to be its least technological: timely and comprehensive discussions with patients as they near death. Without this open conversation about death, patients are traumatized needlessly, leaving their families with the emotional scars of witnessing the hyper-medicalized deaths of their loved ones. I, too, am guilty of sometimes failing to have frank discussions with my patients and their loved ones. As a hospitalist — a physician specializing in the treatment of sick patients in a hospital setting — I am reminded of this as I witness a handful of the 2.5 million deaths that occur in this country each year.

People simply don't know death in its twenty-first-century guise. Fifty years ago, most people died at home surrounded by their loved ones; today, most deaths occur in health care institutions where patients are surrounded by strangers. By most accounts, this transformation of death from a natural process occurring at home to a medicalized event taking place outside of the home has been disastrous. The blitz of medical interventions that accompany modern death is difficult for many to imagine because the majority of deaths take place out of sight, hidden behind the walls of hospitals and nursing homes. And the bowdlerized images of CPR and other interventions routinely shown on television and in the movies do little to inform people of what medical care in hospitals at the end of life truly looks like. Much of the medical care that is delivered at the end of life to patients in the advanced stages of a disease would largely be rejected if patients and families had a better sense of what it involved. When we reach for the latest and greatest in medical interventions without understanding whether the benefits are marginal or simply prolong the suffering at the end of life, the result is that many of us die today with tubes emanating from every orifice and cracked ribs and punctured lungs from the rigors of CPR, surrounded by people we've never met but who will likely be the last ones we see in this world.

In this era of high-technology medicine, people have come to see cutting-edge advances and medical miracles as the norm. Each new advance, however, pushes the boundary between life and death into murky territory where patients are largely bewildered and the goals are less clear.

Clearly, burdensome medical interventions that cause profound pain and suffering have saved millions of lives when performed in patients who have a treatable illness with a reasonable prognosis. When the benefits are great, most people are willing to tolerate a good deal of physical pain and suffering. A triple bypass, for example, involves sawing and cracking your chest open, followed by months of rigorous physical therapy. A bone marrow biopsy involves a rigid needle the length of your hand being screwed into the back of your hip bone as liquid marrow is sucked out of your bone. Many patients are willing to undergo these procedures because the longer-term benefits are both clear and demonstrable. In other words, the pain is worth the effort since there is a good chance that the procedure will help. But the risk-benefit calculus is far more difficult and uncertain for patients with a terminal illness, for whom the burdens are great and the benefits minimal.

The dizzying array of decisions that must be made as people with a serious illness approach the end of their lives is part and parcel of a modern American death. What people need most on this journey is not the promise of the next new technology but rather a guide to help navigate this dark forest in which they will undoubtedly find themselves. People need doctors who are capable of explaining new technologies with the accompanying risks and benefits, and discussing whether those technologies would truly benefit them. The health care system is teeming with brilliant scientists, but there is a dearth of effective communicators and advocates.

Over the last few decades, clinicians who are experts in navigating hospitals and complex medical interventions have emerged. These professionals usually reside in departments of palliative care. Unfortunately, they are few in number and receive only a sliver of the resources needed to do their jobs well. Patients pay the price for this shortsightedness and lack of funding, and in order to address the scale of the problem, all doctors, not just palliative care doctors, should be highly trained communicators who insist on discussions with patients about medical care at the end of life.

The Conversation stems from my belief that one toxic side effect of the extraordinary progress that has been made in medical technology is the assault of medical interventions at the very end of life. The first, necessary step toward a remedy lies with a return to the oldest tool in medicine's proverbial black bag: talking with patients about their wishes for how they want to live their remaining time. If the health care system slows the technological juggernaut enough for doctors to explain fully to seriously ill patients the options for medical care as the end of life approaches — including the choice to forgo countless interventions in advanced illness, if that is indeed what is desired — then patients can truly choose how to spend the remainder of their lives.

Among the questions that all of us, as future patients, need to consider and discuss with family, close friends, and our doctors are the following:

- What kinds of things are important to you in your life?
- If you were not able to do the activities you enjoy, are there any medical

21

treatments that would be too much?

- What fears do you have about getting sick or medical care?
- Do you have any spiritual, religious, philosophical, or cultural beliefs that guide you when you make medical decisions?
- If you had to choose between living longer or having a higher quality of life, which would you pick?
- How important is it for you to be at home when you die?

Some people will leave end-of-life decisions to their personal physicians and other experts, without questioning them. Some, like Lillian Badakian, will choose to pursue any possible remedy, no matter how extreme, painful, or experimental, in an effort to stave off the ravages of disease, the trauma of serious accident or injury, or just the gentle unwinding of life functions that accompanies old age. Others will opt for hospice care to ensure comfort, a sense of community, and access to family and friends as the end approaches. The success of this essential conversation about end-of-life care lies not in the individual path chosen but rather in the active and fully informed participation of the patient and family members. In other words, these discussions empower patients to receive whatever end-of-life medical care they wish.

The Conversation explores the lives of seven seriously ill patients who experienced very different deaths, each hinging on whether or not a doctor had a discussion with the patient before he or she could no longer make a decision. In the case of those people who did not have the benefit of discussing their options, the stories of their end-of-life care exhibit the neglect that deeply permeates the U.S. health care system. They offer a glimpse into the hidden hospital world that defines how many Americans die.

By exploring the experiences of people whose deaths were improved by discussing their preferences ahead of time, the reader is offered a template, a way to make sure that the care delivered at the end of life is consistent with his or her wishes. Yet, sometimes words alone are not enough to have The Conversation successfully, so the reader is also introduced to the latest in video resources that offer a realistic picture of medical care and accurate depictions of what medical technology can and cannot do. Empowering patients with videos to supplement verbal discussions with doctors and nurses further educates people so they can die as they wish.

As a doctor I, too, have prolonged the dying process needlessly. Inflicting harm and suffering on dying patients is a heavy burden that I reluctantly acknowledge. It is a source of great unease as I confront the mortality of my loved ones — and, someday, my own death. At first, my medical training and experience as a young doctor impeded me from understanding the role of death in life, but I gradually arrived at the undeniable reality for physicians: To doctor patients is to learn how not to die.

This thought haunted me for some time until I realized that many of my colleagues had similar views. Although we had spent years learning the complexities of medical physiology and transforming ourselves into technological wizards, we failed to hone our skills as physician-communicators — that is, as professionals who valued talking to our patients and engaging them in honest discussions. We answered the call of medicine in order to do good, yet the overwhelming majority of us treat patients with serious illness in a manner we would never want for our loved ones, or even for ourselves.

It is my profound hope that this book galvanizes patients, families, and doctors to establish a new standard of care. If a doctor doesn't initiate the crucial discussion about end-of-life care, *The Conversation* anchors patients and their preferences at the core of medical care by emboldening them to start the dialogue. Patients can drive change by having greater knowledge of their options, while doctors can drive change by communicating and advocating for those choices. Doctors have good reason to be the catalysts of change; every doctor knows that in the end, we all find ourselves on the patient's side of the stethoscope.

CHAPTER ONE:
MY MEDICAL ODYSSEY

As the child of Greek immigrants, I was fed centuries' worth of Greek classics: tragedy, epic poetry, and philosophy. Every day I read about a fateful twist in Aeschylus' tragedies, another adventurous wandering in wily Odysseus' journey back to Ithaca, or an ironic passage by one of history's great gadflies, Socrates. But the books that consumed me, the ones I kept reading and rereading, were the ones on philosophy. Plato and Aristotle were my constant companions. They seemed to ask the really tough questions about virtue and excellence, about ideals and community, about the good life — and the good death. As Socrates argued, philosophy is, ultimately, a preparation for death.

A good life? A good death? Not exactly Saturday-morning-cartoon material. How did one answer the big questions about life and death? How did philosophy lead to wisdom and knowledge about these issues? Such questions kept reverberating in my mind throughout my adolescence, as if they were being debated by the grumbling Greek expats who frequented my parents' Manhattan diner, and not by another chorus of Greeks in Athens, 2,500 years earlier. I was fascinated by those questions, and when I entered college in the late 1980s, it was only natural that I declared myself a philosophy major.

When I wasn't reading as a teenager, I was waiting tables at the diner, where I picked up some of my family's knack for cooking. Despite working long hours and saving every nickel and dime, my working-class family could barely afford the astronomical tuition of a college education, let alone the additional money to pay for books and school supplies. I passed on the minimum-wage job cleaning dormitory bathrooms offered by the college financial aid office and instead searched for a more lucrative opportunity. "Wanted: Personal Cook for Emeritus Professor and His Wife." I tore the classified ad from the student newspaper and called the professor to get more details. It turned out that his wife was ill, and they were in need of someone to help prepare meals. I headed out on my secondhand bicycle to the professor's home, only a five-minute ride from campus.

Benedict C. Stone IV was a campus legend. For forty years he'd taught the introductory course on political philosophy, and he was often spotted in his printed flannel smoking jacket walking the tree-lined trails on campus as he pulled on his pipe. Patty, his wife, played the traditional role of the academic's wife: hosting scrumptious French-inspired dinners for students and cocktail parties for his faculty colleagues and commenting on his work. When she wasn't preparing an haute-cuisine dessert, she could be found on the living room couch with a cigarette in one hand and a pencil in the other as she fine-tuned Benedict's latest opus.

But now everything had changed. Patty was dying from emphysema. She could no longer prepare her favorite French meals. They hired me to cook all their dinners and so had to settle for the Greek-inspired fare that I had picked up at the diner. I would attend classes during the day and then jump on my bike and ride off to their home by afternoon to prepare their evening meal.

All the years of smoking those dainty Virginia Slims had finally taken their toll on Patty. "It was de rigueur back then. 'You've come a long way, baby.' All the ladies smoked," she would tell me. She could barely walk a few steps without suffocating in breathlessness. An oxygen tank was always by her side.

One sunny late afternoon as I was putting the finishing touches on a rosemary-crusted roasted lamb, I heard coughing. It was coming from Patty's bedroom. She had a typical smoker's cough, lots of phlegm and always gurgling, but this time her cough was different. It had a deeper, visceral quality.

The professor heard it as well and we both ran to her bedroom. Patty could barely breathe. One could no longer make out the embroidery on her white handkerchief; it was soaked with blood. Her once pink lips were tinged with blue and her nails, a dusky gray. She lifted her sunken eyes and looked at her husband as if to say "Not to worry, sweetheart." But how could he not worry? She was gasping for air, each breath a struggle. She was literally suffocating to death right before our eyes.

"Do you think we should give her some more of the medicine to ease her breathing and make her comfortable? Should we call an ambulance and go to the hospital?" the professor asked me, his once sturdy voice relegated to a whisper. I was in shock, frozen and unresponsive. I had never seen someone gasping for air or so much blood.

"What should we do?" he continued. "I never expected this so soon. Patty and I never talked about this. I just don't know anymore. What do you think, Angelo?"

I couldn't tell who was suffering more at that moment, this giant of a man, at a loss and tearing up, or his blue-lipped wife. Years later as a doctor, I would replay this scene over and over as I saw patients' family members despair at the impending death of their wife, mother, father, or brother. Disease may invade the bodies of patients, but the experience of illness devastates all those around them. Suffering demands that others bear witness, and family members are assigned front-row seats.

Luckily, within a few minutes, Patty's coughing subsided on its own. The pink returned to her lips, and the choking, gurgling sounds gradually decreased. She fell asleep as the professor held her hand, tears streaming down his cheeks. We were all given a reprieve.

I headed back to the dormitory. Although final exams were approaching, I could not find the mental focus to study. My thoughts kept returning to Patty's panting breath and the blotches of blood on her handkerchief.

And the professor's questions echoed in my mind: What did I think? What is a good death? Dying at home? Dying in a hospital? Choking to death? Dying peacefully?

Months after Patty's death I pondered the difference between thinking about death and suffering and witnessing it. Learning about death (and life) through clinical experience would be the necessary ingredient to a proper understanding. The semester following after Patty's death, my interest turned from philosophy to medicine.

Over the years as a physician, I have accompanied hundreds of people on that final journey. I am no longer frozen by a bloody handkerchief or a loved one's grief. And the single most important lesson that I have learned is the same one that I absorbed when Professor Stone turned to me in panic and despair: In order to make decisions about life and death, people need to know more about life's final chapter. In order to experience a good death, we must do more than think about death and suffering: We need to talk about it openly.

Some of my classmates entered medical school aspiring to combat infectious diseases that persist as scourges of the developing world, while others savored the challenge of performing the most dexterous operations.

And some were pursuing a prestigious career or financial security. I entered medical school hoping to understand what it meant for patients to be sick and dying, and to prepare them for their journey.

My proclivity has always been to talk with my patients, to hear about their experiences, and to understand their hopes and fears. But I soon discovered that talking with patients is not a priority in my profession. In fact, it is often ignored entirely. There are too many other things to learn: ventricular fibrillation and atrio-ventricular nodal reentrant rhythms; tailored genetic therapies and recently discovered genetic mutations; acid-base disturbances and cholesterol-lowering medications. The onslaught of laboratory results and the mining of patient data points leave little space for doctors to consider their patients' stories. Unfortunately, by barring patients from treatment decisions, doctors inevitably lose their moral compass. One patient taught me this important lesson a long time ago.

Taras Skripchenko was a living part of American history. As I later found out from his local priest, Taras was an ethnic Ukrainian who had emigrated to the United States from the Soviet Union as an adolescent. He was one of the lucky few who escaped the chaos that took over during the months before World War II in what is present-day Ukraine. Taras wanted to start over, to rewrite the opening chapters of his life. At eighteen, he found a new home in a Ukrainian enclave in one of the mining towns of Appalachia and quickly found labor in the coal mines. For years, he led a life of unremitting physical toil, working twelve-hour shifts, six days a week.

Unfortunately for Taras, a lot of the detritus from smashing coal dug its way deep into the lining of his lungs, plugging the airways. It would also plant the creeping cancer that would devastate him decades later. This once hulking mine worker had dwindled to a mere whisper of his former muscular self. This frail, bed-bound seventy-eight-year-old with inoperable lung cancer was admitted to my medical service during my first year of residency training. Slowly suffocating to death, he experienced both transient moments of hallucinatory joy and unconscious yet peaceful somnolence on Eliot 7, the oncology ward.

Taras was too confused to have a lucid conversation and lacked family members to guide his decision-making, so his medical plan was the default approach for all patients: Do everything possible to keep him alive. Taras's oncologists had failed to speak with him earlier in the course of his disease about what level of medical care he desired when the cancer inevitably advanced. I am not sure why this discussion had not occurred; most likely they had not wanted to scare him. Even today, some oncologists are hesitant to discuss medical care with patients in the advanced stages of cancer out of fear that they will dash any hope the patient clings to, despite the extensive medical research that indicates many patients do, in fact, want to talk about these topics with their physicians.

In one large study published in 2008 by the *Journal of the American Medical Association,* a group of oncologists from the Dana-Farber Cancer Institute in Boston studied the influence of having end-of-life discussions with 332 patients suffering from advanced cancer. The researchers found no evidence of emotional distress or psychiatric illness in patients who had end-of-life discussions with their physicians. Patients who did not have a similar exchange with their physicians were more likely to have a lesser quality of life than patients who did. In addition, the loved ones of patients who did not discuss options with their doctors were more likely to be depressed.

Because Taras had no family members available, I sought guidance from his local priest. Unfortunately, the general contours of Taras's life were all that were available. No one knew his preferences for medical care, and he had not completed a living will or other advance directive stating his wishes. Additionally, there were many details to gather before what doctors call the "goals of care" could be planned. A patient's goals of care serve as a larger picture for the medical team, so they can consider issues beyond the patient's immediate ones. Despite my efforts to come up with a plan for Taras, I knew that his cancer surely had a plan of its own. Doctors can fool themselves into thinking that they are in charge, even when disease and pathology are in the driver's seat. Frequently, we are only along for the ride.

Taras was dying. I knew it and the nurses knew it. But as far as the medical team was concerned, Taras was a "full code," because he had not requested a Do Not Resuscitate (DNR) order. In today's hyper-medicalized world, doctors, nurses, and hospitals all work under the assumption that, unless clearly stated in advance, a patient in crisis is full code no matter what. If his heart or lungs stopped working, we would attempt CPR and place him on a breathing machine. In short, we were prepared to do everything possible to keep him alive.

I was worried about Taras; his breathing had become more erratic, more labored. I decided to swing by his room that evening before heading home. Surprisingly, his heart rate, blood pressure, and oxygen saturation were stable. He looked slightly better and had a little more pink in his cheeks. Relieved and exhausted from the long day, I paged the overnight resident to meet me in the cafeteria to review my list of patients before I signed out for the night.

The overnight doctor was a senior resident named Edward, and I was glad an experienced resident was on call that night. I told the resident to keep a close watch on Taras Skripchenko on Eliot 7. "He is a Ukrainian gentleman originally from the U.S.S.R. who worked in the coal mines of Appalachia. About eight months ago he began having a cough, saw his primary care doctor, who ordered a chest X-ray —"

"Stop right there," he said. "Start again. Start with initials, and then in one line give me the pertinent info. Less is more. I have thirty other patients to cover tonight." When a resident is responsible for thirty patients at night, too many personal details can muddle one's thinking.

"T. S. is a seventy-eight-year-old male patient with metastatic lung cancer who presented with shortness of breath and delirium," I said. "He's really sick."

For the overnight resident, personal details were extraneous to the task at hand, which was to make sure no patient died on his watch. In today's medical speak, patients are pared down to age, gender, and disease: sixty-five-year-old female with atypical chest pain; eighty-nine-year-old male with acute kidney injury. The use of initials serves the pragmatic purpose of differentiating patients. For the medical staff, a patient's diagnosis, treatment, and prognosis could be summarized by two letters.

Modern medicine can be dehumanizing, and the first step in that process is to remove all the individualized details — to obliterate personhood and replace it with patient-hood, where only the medical details matter. This was one of the earliest lessons hammered into me as a young physician. At first I thought it was to protect patient confidentiality, since physicians often discussed patients in the elevators or cafeteria within earshot of visiting patients' families who would certainly not appreciate hearing about their loved one's medical status while ordering a BLT at the cafeteria. I quickly learned, however, that using patients' initials had more to do with emotional distance. To confront and endure the deaths and suffering of so many patients, doctors seek to distance themselves from their patients, to reduce them to little more than anonymous bodies defined by their conditions.

"Code Blue, Eliot Seven! Code Blue, Eliot Seven!" Edward and I sprinted toward the oncology ward. Racing through the obstacle course of stretchers and patients, we finally arrived, out of breath, at Taras's room. I was always taught to hope for the best but prepare for the worst before walking into a patient's room, but it's not always clear how to define the worst.

The gathered nurses who had ordered the Code Blue had already started CPR. I clumsily jammed my hands into a pair of rubber gloves and joined the ritual, relieving one of the nurses doing chest compressions, which is far more physically demanding — and brutal — than what is portrayed on television. My clasped hands pressed hard against Taras's frail chest, and all I could hear and feel were the cracking of his ribs with practically each chest compression. The rhythmic pumping on his chest eerily emitted a coarse, Velcro-like sound.

Edward stood at the foot of the bed and took charge, directing what was likely to be Taras's passage from life. "Continue chest compressions, and let's secure an airway. Get that heart monitor and pads ready in case we need to shock. This is straight out of the playbook, folks." Even as adrenaline was coursing through everyone's veins, we remained a unified body, each part performing its assigned role. I was in charge of compressions, someone else was pumping air into his lungs with a green breathing bag, and another was administering lifesaving drugs. The team was well trained and prepared for just such moments.

"Please stop compressions, and let's check for a pulse," Edward calmly instructed. I was amazed at how cool and collected he remained in the presence of impending death. I searched for a pulse on Taras's neck. Any fat had melted away long ago, and all I could feel was cartilage and windpipe. It is an eerie feeling, sliding bloody gloved fingers along the skin, searching for signs of life. Shockingly, I found only a "thready" pulse, one that lacked vigor.

Taras was stabilized. I do not remember how long it took, or what medicines we gave; these details are a blur now. But the outcome remains clear. He was connected to a breathing machine and had a pulse with a normal rhythm. The team had saved the patient, and now it was time to transfer him to the intensive care unit. I never liked calling it that. The whole hospital gave intensive care regardless of where the patient was located. But the monitoring in the intensive care unit — the ICU — was more extensive, as were the interventions available there: powerful medications that helped the heartbeat, ventilators, ultrasound machines, and even a dialysis suite.

Edward and I bundled Taras and his machines onto a gurney and navigated the labyrinth of hallways to the elevator. We also carried with us all the necessary medications and syringes in case something unexpected happened along the way. We squeezed into the narrow elevator as the doors closed. I kept my hand on Taras's carotid artery, making sure to feel for a pulse, until I realized he no longer had one. Despite the electric waves on the heart monitor, his heart was not beating properly. Taras was almost dead.

There was no space alongside the gurney so I jumped on, straddled him, and started performing chest compressions. Edward and I quickly ran through the most common complications that might cause Taras not to have a pulse. Perhaps he had blood surrounding his heart. Cancer can spread to just about anywhere, and lung cancer sometimes invades the thin sac around the heart, known as the pericardium. The pericardium typically serves as a protective shell around the heart and as a sheath so that when the heart pumps it doesn't bump into surrounding blood vessels and bones. However, when cancer invades the pericardium, blood and fluid seep into the sac and limit the space around the vigorously pumping heart muscle, making it all but impossible for the heart to fill properly. If the heart cannot fill with blood, it cannot pump out blood to the rest of the body. This is called cardiac tamponade, from the French for obstruction, *tamponnade.* To get the heart pumping properly, a doctor must perform pericardiocentesis by sticking a large needle into the patient's chest and drawing the fluid out.

We needed to move fast.

"Do you feel comfortable doing this?" Edward asked. I told him that I had performed the procedure on a cadaver in anatomy class but had only seen one on a patient. "See one. Do one. Teach one. Here's your chance on a warm body," he rejoined, as the elevator doors opened to a crowd of nurses ready to wheel the patient toward the ICU.

I descended from the gurney. Edward handed me a large syringe attached to a needle the length of my ring finger. "Time is not on our side, so let's just do it," he told me. Outside of the elevator, in the middle of the hallway, I stared at the needle. My hands were shaking, not surprising since I was about to poke around a man's heart with a needle. During an emergency pericardiocentesis, you don't know how deep to slide the needle into the body in order to draw out the fluid from the sac surrounding the heart. Every body is different: Some are fatter than others and some are more muscular than fat. Pointing the needle at a 30-degree angle toward the left nipple, my anatomical landmark for the heart, I pierced his skin just below the sternum on the xiphoid process, a cartilaginous extension that is shaped like a sharply pointed spear. Xiphoid comes from the Greek word *xiphos,* for sharp sword.

I carefully pushed the needle through the skin, minimal fat, and atrophied muscle, hoping to see a rush of blood-tinged fluid into the plastic syringe; if I saw bright red blood flash back into the syringe, the needle

43

had gone too deep and into the heart itself. Millimeter by millimeter I continued pushing, simultaneously pulling back on the syringe, hoping for fluid. No luck. The tremulousness in my hands worsened and beads of sweat trickled down my forehead, falling onto the syringe. I advanced the needle a little more, but before I knew it, the syringe had filled with bright-colored blood, likely from inside the heart. Maybe we were wrong about the cardiac tamponade, or perhaps my technique was faulty.

I pulled the needle out and tried again. And again. And again. By the fourth time, I gave up. Residents are usually allowed three strikes before being asked to stop; Edward gave me a fourth since this was my patient. I probably should have stopped after the third. Taras's rib cage had become a pincushion from all my attempts.

Edward gave an additional salvo of commands to the ICU nurses: "One milligram of epi, followed by chest compressions, followed by more stacked doses of epi. Get the IV meds ready in case this is a blood clot in the lungs. Let's wheel him to the unit." The nurses gathered around the gurney in the middle of the hospital hallway as we made our way to the ICU. The fresh entourage of physicians there was eager to receive Taras.

As soon as we entered the ICU, Edward filled in the medical team as they took over, using the ultrasound machine to get a better look at the sac surrounding Taras's heart and rapidly inserting a needle to remove the viscous blood-tinged liquid. It was just under 100 milliliters (about a quarter of a soda can), which may not sound like a lot, but only a few tablespoons of liquid surrounding the heart were the difference between life and death. Taras's once flailing heart could beat again. He had a pulse.

It was late in the evening. Taras's care was now being managed by the ICU team, so Edward and I headed back to the cafeteria to grab some coffee. After every Code Blue, the team is expected to review what transpired. It is a ritualized moment to grapple with the trauma surrounding a full-on code. It was too late to gather the others, so Edward and I decided to carry out the debriefing on our own.

Debriefings are always difficult moments as each of us dials down the rapid pace of a Code Blue to digest the events that have just transpired. We sat quietly for a few minutes until Edward blurted out, "Well, I guess that's one less patient for you to see tomorrow." Neither of us laughed, but it did break the ice. We reviewed the running of the code, how each team member had performed his or her duties. We replayed each of the interventions I had performed and discussed how I could sharpen my technique the next time I poked a needle toward someone's heart.

Silence settled again once the routine items were out of the way, but there was more to be said.

"We just completed a by-the-book code, but I wonder if we did the right thing," I said, needing to tell Edward what was on my mind. Perhaps it was because I was a young doctor and I had not yet been numbed to the brutal experience of caring for hundreds of patients. I hoped Edward, a more seasoned doctor, would have a better perspective.

"We did exactly what we were taught to do, everything was by the book. Look, this is the system. We have a job to do," he said, but I could see a slight unease in his face, a hint of upheaval.

We both knew that something was not right. "I can't believe we just did all that to a man who has one foot in the grave," I pushed, not mincing my words. "Would he have wanted any of this? Would you have wanted any of this? Would you do this to your dad? Something is wrong with a system that puts terminal cancer patients through torture." Edward put a hand on my shoulder. "It's going to be all right. You're still new at this. You'll get used to it. Get some sleep and page me tomorrow morning when you come back to work."

Get used to it? Is one supposed to get used to this?

Over the next two days, Edward and I visited Taras every few hours in the ICU. He was no longer our patient, but we could not let go of him, either. By the following morning he had a tube or catheter in almost every part of his body, for a grand total of eight plastic intrusions, including an endotracheal tube (lungs), two central intravenous lines (veins), an arterial line, a nasogastric tube (stomach), a foley catheter (bladder), a rectal trumpet tube, and a tube placed in the sac of his heart to drain fluid. The cardiologists and cardiothoracic surgeons had decided to fix the problem of cardiac tamponade by cutting a hole, a cardiac window, in the wall of the pericardium so that fluid could not build up and constrict the heart. Taras was "fixed."

Doctors like to tackle problems and fix them. And it is truly amazing what modern medicine has achieved in a relatively brief span of time. Can't breathe? We can fix that with breathing machines. Have an infection in the blood? We can fix that with powerful antibiotics. Have some fluid around the heart? We can even fix that by drawing it off with a needle or cutting a hole into the pericardial sac that surrounds the heart. The tougher issue, however, is when to recognize that the small fixes do not change the larger picture, to recognize that fixing specific problems may not fix the whole patient.

This is medicine's version of not seeing the forest for the trees. The cardiologists and cardiothoracic surgeons had repaired Taras's heart, but what benefit was this to him? Could he go on living in a meaningful way? Doctors always search for the next fix, but we need to know when to use — or not use — our growing tool kit of fixes. If no one asks the critically ill patient whether or not he or she would even want these risky procedures that offer marginal benefits, if any, then doctors just keep on trying more interventions.

Taras's heart had stopped three more times, and, miraculously, the ICU team had brought him back each time. But, not surprisingly, a patient in the late stages of terminal advanced cancer succumbed to his disease. Whatever the next new fix is, nature eventually takes her inexorable course. Taras died forty-eight hours after the Code Blue.

Americans receive some of the best health care money can buy; they also experience some of the worst deaths in the developed world. Complications from life-prolonging interventions, poor continuity of care between hospitals and clinics, and medical errors are some of the reasons for this unfortunate fact. However, the primary reason we experience such horrible deaths is doctors' failure to openly discuss medical care with seriously ill patients.

Taras was the lucky beneficiary of the latest cutting-edge technological breakthroughs in cancer research, the most skilled cardiologists and cardiothoracic surgeons on Earth, and the most sophisticated medical care delivered at one of the country's best hospitals. Modern medicine is founded on the conviction that technology will conquer all, including death. From the first day of medical school through the last day of residency and fellowship, the promise of technology is implanted in every new doctor's DNA. Breakthrough discoveries that are only read about in class soon become the next new thing by the time young doctors finish training. Taras would have been dead months earlier had he not received the latest round of chemotherapy or antibiotics fighting superbugs.

But how might his last few months have been different?

From the very first primary care doctor who ordered a chest X-ray when Taras had a cough, to the last doctor who admitted him to the hospital prior to his death, each one undoubtedly asked him a battery of questions regarding his medicines, allergies, and family history of cancer. Yet, it appeared that no one had inquired about his wishes regarding end-of-life care.

Talking to patients is given short shrift in medical training. The focus of medical education is on technology and treatments; medicine is about doing, not talking. Communicating with patients, especially about end-of-life care, usually takes a backseat. If the ten years of my undergraduate and graduate medical education were plotted onto a single calendar year, the amount of time I spent learning to talk with patients about medical care would likely last a single day. The other 364 are spent learning about everything else in medicine.

When I completed residency, in order to become a board-certified physician I was required to prove my competence with inserting central line catheters, leading

Code Blues, performing lumbar punctures, drawing blood, and obtaining arterial blood gas samples. But not a single senior physician needed to certify that I could actually speak to patients about medical care. Ironically, I have not inserted a central line or performed many of the other tested procedures since residency, but I speak to patients and families daily.

Much has changed since my training days, and for the better. More medical schools are introducing communication training into their curricula. Students attend small group sessions on how to talk with patients and practice role-playing with actors who play the part of patients. Two schools in particular, the University of Rochester School of Medicine in Rochester, New York, and the Icahn School of Medicine at Mount Sinai in New York City, have taken the lead in integrating communication training into the fabric of their medical schools.

In Rochester, medical students are assigned seriously ill patients from primary care clinics early in their training. Students then make home visits to meet their patients and over the course of their visits ask the tough questions that no one asked Taras: What makes life worth living? What fears do you have about medical care? Are there circumstances in which you would find life not worth living? Do you have spiritual or religious beliefs that help guide your decisions? Rochester medical students are taught to ask these questions alongside the more traditional questions that doctors ask patients regarding symptoms, medications, and drug allergies. Thus, talking about end-of-life care is given equal weight to more routine medical questions and becomes ingrained in the habits of young physicians.

At Mount Sinai, all medical students are required to spend a week on rotation with the school's nationally recognized palliative care team, which is led by Dr. Diane Meier, arguably the country's leader in the field. Students participate in providing clinical care to some of the sickest hospitalized patients in the country, learning firsthand about patient autonomy, health care proxies, Do Not Resuscitate orders, ventilator withdrawal, the risk-benefit ratios of medical treatments, and how to lead discussions with patients and families about their goals of medical care. These clinical exposures to end-of-life communication are potent emotional experiences that are seared into medical students' developing identities as doctors. Dr. Meier describes such real student-patient interactions as "the difference between watching a movie about war and being in war."

Yet Rochester and Mount Sinai are in the minority in integrating communication training into the medical school curriculum. In 2008, a group of Dartmouth researchers surveyed all 128 U.S. medical schools regarding offerings in "Palliative and Hospice Care." Of the forty-eight medical schools that responded to the survey, only fourteen had a required course and only nine had a mandatory rotation on the subject. Seven schools offered an elective course and fourteen had an optional rotation for students that were interested in the topic. The researchers concluded that only a small fraction of U.S. medical schools required training in communicating with patients with advanced, incurable conditions.

After medical school, most practical training for communicating with patients takes place during residency. In order to maintain accreditation today, residency programs must certify that residents can indeed communicate with patients and families. Programs must have a curriculum to teach communication skills to trainees, usually a handful of lectures on communication throughout the duration of residency. Those residents interested in more robust training can take additional electives in palliative care.

Although these are notable advances in residency education, other changes in medical training countervail these valiant efforts. The amount of information that trainees must master before graduating residency has exploded in the last decade. The technological advances and treatment modalities with which residents must be familiar are mind-boggling. I am often reminded of this when my residents update me on the latest medical advances. Concurrent with the explosion of medical knowledge is the fact that residents are now limited to no more than eighty hours per week, which still constitutes a brutal workweek. More information is squeezed — crammed, really — into less time. Perhaps, if we imagine a medical education compressed into one year again, that training now lasts two or three days. That is not sufficient.

Not surprisingly, it is easier to train some doctors than others to improve their communication skills. Some medical students and residents are simply better communicators, more comfortable expressing and listening to others. The same can be said of the ability to conduct physical exams or to memorize medications. However, there is one significant difference among these aptitudes: Medical schools place far more importance on the capacity of applicants to show expertise in scientific reasoning, mathematical skills, and memorization at the expense of the ability to communicate.

Standard premed requirements include years of scientific study in biology, chemistry, physics, and organic chemistry, among others — and bonus points are given to those applicants who enroll in the most challenging science classes. But few are the medical schools that value classes in English studies, rhetoric, philosophy, communication, or other related "soft" disciplines. When a medical school class consists of future doctors who have shown aptitude in memorizing the Krebs cycle but have difficulty communicating bad news to patients, is it any surprise that brief communication training is not effective? Perhaps in the near future, medical schools can implement selection criteria that value the ability to talk with patients and families alongside the many other qualifications for young doctors.

Talking to patients and families is hard

work. It is stressful, uncomfortable, and easy to shunt aside in favor of other pressing duties. And it takes practice, lots of it. Surgeons cannot conduct surgery without supervision until they have completed a certain number of supervised surgeries and proven their ability to perform. Yet when it comes to talking with patients about end-of-life care, doctors rarely acknowledge the skill and practice needed to perform one of the hardest "procedures" of all: having The Conversation with patients and families. Unfortunately, this short-sightedness results in patients' lives that end with bad deaths.

Taras Skripchenko died fifteen years ago. I have since witnessed hundreds of deaths, but his — which I experienced during the formative experience of medical residency — haunted me for the first decade of my life as a young physician. So, too, did that late-night conversation with Edward, as we both struggled to make sense of the drama that had just unfolded in front of us. Today, I am a full-fledged medical doctor, a senior physician, and teacher of others, yet I still think about Taras each time I meet a new patient.

CHAPTER TWO:
"DO EVERYTHING"

Patients are not the only victims of bad deaths; their families suffer as well. Taras didn't have any relatives to advocate on his behalf, but generally patients who are too ill to make a decision count on their families to do so for them. Few patients have actually discussed their preferences for end-of-life care with their families, and in the absence of this information, family members are forced to make difficult choices under duress, as they battle grief and other complex emotions. There is no guarantee they can protect the patient from a health care system that promotes taking every possible measure to keep a person alive. In fact, they can unknowingly enable it, as the family of Assunta Antonia Bruno did.

"How was your night?" I asked the overnight physician before I took over for the day.

"Not bad," she reported. "Just one patient for you, but she's a train wreck: A.B. — 84-year-old female with advanced Alzheimer's. She was a late-night transfer from surgery."

Assunta Antonia Bruno, affectionately known as Nonna (the matriarch), had opened a restaurant in the suburbs of Boston once her three children were of school age; thirteen grandchildren and four great-grandchildren later, the trattoria was a labor of family love. She had been diagnosed with Alzheimer's disease five years earlier, when her daughter noticed that Nonna had forgotten to add the tomatoes to her famous pasta e fagioli (pasta and beans).

Nonna had been in the hospital for weeks. Despite her failing cognitive health and her age, orthopedic surgeons had replaced her hip after a fall and she had suffered numerous complications after the surgery. First pneumonia clogged one of her lungs, almost suffocating her until a tube was inserted down her throat and she was temporarily placed on a breathing machine. Then she developed a blood clot that traveled from her leg to her lungs, requiring a blood thinner to make sure the clot did not spread elsewhere.

During this ordeal, in hopes that Nonna would improve, the family had requested that a feeding tube be inserted as a last-ditch effort to provide her with nourishment. The latest indignity was a serious abdominal skin infection surrounding the site of the feeding tube, which Nonna had inadvertently pulled out while in a state of delirium.

Unfortunately, advanced Alzheimer's disease is a terminal condition. The health care team could address the pneumonia, the clot, and the abdominal infection — all complications after the initial hip replacement — but in the end, Nonna had a terminal condition with no hope for a cure in her lifetime. What seemed like an innocent hip surgery had metamorphosed into a medical nightmare. Nonna had no recollection of the ravages her body had suffered, but her family was painfully aware of this Kafkaesque hyper-medicalized journey.

It was a vertiginous undertaking to keep track of all the particulars of this case. The overnight doctor did an admirable job crystallizing Nonna's medical history in just a few brief moments, giving me the highlights of her stay in the hospital. At the end of her review she added, "I haven't spoken to any of the patient's family members about where we go from here, but I suggest that you have a meeting with them as soon as possible. I gave her antibiotics for the abdominal infection, but the family needs to make a decision about replacing the feeding tube." Nonna was clearly at the tail end of a downward spiral.

Hers was a sad story, but one that I encountered all too often. About a fifth of the patients admitted to the hospital have some form of dementia, a medical term encompassing various disorders associated with loss of memory and other cognitive difficulties that are severe enough to impede a person's ability to function in daily life. Alzheimer's disease is the most common form, accounting for 60 to 80 percent of all cases of dementia. The second most common is vascular dementia, which occurs after a stroke. People with vascular dementia initially present with impaired judgment or the inability to plan steps needed to complete a task, rather than the memory loss associated with Alzheimer's disease. Depending on where in the brain the stroke occurred, different functions are affected. In 2012, there were more than 35 million people in the world living with dementia; it is estimated that there are 7.7 million new cases each year.

The German psychiatrist Alois Alzheimer identified the first case of what would be later known as Alzheimer's disease more than a century ago, yet the disease remains 100 percent incurable and ultimately 100 percent fatal. Despite innovative hypotheses and scores of clinical trials with medicines thought to be promising, the profession still has very little in its arsenal to treat the disease. Equally problematic are misperceptions about the stages of Alzheimer's disease. The public forms its opinion and makes decisions about medical care in Alzheimer's disease in part by the images it sees on television: a confused, elderly grandmother forgetting a name, or a dazed, well-groomed grandfather leaving a heated stove unattended. These are accurate images of Alzheimer's disease, but only in its early stages.

In the first stage of Alzheimer's disease, people have problems with memory that are severe enough to get in the way of everyday activities. In the middle stages, problems with memory, language, and behavior worsen. Patients may leave a boiling kettle on the stove, or be so confused that their spoken language makes no sense. Behavioral changes become more pronounced and many middle-stage sufferers become suspicious or paranoid. The advanced stages of Alzheimer's include severe changes in memory, language, and behavior. These patients may not recognize their loved ones. They say or understand only a few words. They cannot do the most basic things such as eating, speaking, walking, washing themselves, or going to the bathroom, and they often push away the caregivers who try to help them. It is like the progression of a baby growing into a toddler, only in reverse.

The irony of advanced Alzheimer's disease is that although it untangles the connections in the mind, it leaves other vital organs like the heart intact. What kills you in the end is not Alzheimer's disease, but the consequences of the associated bodily deterioration as the mind shrivels: an infection in the urine, for example; or food trapped in the lungs; or a wound to the buttocks that has developed from immobility. Many people with advanced Alzheimer's disease require more care than their families can provide, and, like my eighty-four-year-old patient, they reside in nursing home communities across the country, tucked away in nondescript brick buildings.

The family meeting was scheduled for later that evening when Nonna's loved ones could convene at the hospital. I wanted to make sure to review all of her medical records beforehand, learning the details of every procedure, from the hip replacement to the feeding tube placement. Little did I know that her medical records were as long as a small encyclopedia divided into numerous volumes and yet completely disorganized. The seemingly only common element among the scores of pages was the name at the top of each page, Assunta Antonia Bruno.

That evening, when I arrived at Nonna's room for the family discussion, I was expecting to meet one or at most two relatives — perhaps a daughter who was particularly close or a nephew who had a special liking for his aunt. I was not expecting a chorus of twenty relatives, which, as I was immediately informed, comprised only half of the family. The others were hard at work at the family's restaurant. Present were Annunziata, the only daughter and the spokesperson for the family; Antonino, the younger of Nonna's two sons; eight grandchildren with all eight of their spouses; and two great-grandchildren. Each face betrayed the torment of the decisions that lay ahead, but it was clear that Annunziata, the firstborn, was the matriarch-in-waiting.

I decided to move the meeting from the cramped quarters of Nonna's room to one of the large conference rooms down the hall. Family meetings are part information session and part confession. Fleshing out the particulars of the patient's disease is not the challenge. The hard part is listening to the family's fears, hopes, and, sometimes, their resentments. Although each family member is likely to feel all of these mixed emotions, they do not necessarily share their thoughts with one another. And when decisions regarding the end of life need to be made, it's critical that the patient's loved ones communicate their feelings.

Nonna had lost the capacity to make decisions on her own years earlier, and her family had already made many on her behalf: hip surgery, blood thinners, and intubation. There are almost always at least two paths one can take at the end of life, and even though they eventually meet, helping families choose for a loved one can be unsettling. Seeking guidance from families is a tricky business, especially when simmering tensions erupt. The doctor may unknowingly enter a family drama that has been playing out for years, and sometimes even over the course of a lifetime. I never know what to expect during such family meetings, so I often begin with the most innocuous of questions: "Tell me about your loved one. What was your mother like before all this?"

"Mama was all about one thing: cooking." Annunziata proceeded to give me a crash course on pasta e fagioli and detailed Nonna's cooking techniques. She then moved on to the etymology of her mother's name: Assunta Antonia had been born on August 15, the same day as the Assumption of the Virgin Mary. Her father, a Sicilian tomato farmer, had prayed to Saint Anthony of Padua, the patron saint of women unable to conceive, to grant him a child. He hoped for a son to help him in the fields, and he planned to name the boy Anthony to honor the saint. His wish for a child was granted, but his wife gave birth to a daughter, not a son. In Catholicism, Mary trumps Anthony, so he named his daughter Assunta (Italian for Assumption) and added the feminized Antonia to cover all his bases. No one interrupted; they sat and listened in rapt attention to each detail of the revered Nonna's life.

I also listened carefully, for the details of patients' lives are fascinating. I had lost my appreciation of their personal stories during medical school and residency. When one is overwhelmed and exhausted by the long hours and grueling demands of a modern medical education, it is easy to overlook the particulars of patients' lives in favor of understanding their diseases. Who had time to learn about Sicilian cooking methods and Catholic rituals when arterial blood pressures and metabolic disturbances needed fixing? I usually tried to justify my lack of attention to personal details by reasoning that patients came to hospitals for technical expertise, not consolation.

While caring for more and more patients, I began to realize, however, that patients and their families came to hospitals not only for technical expertise, but also to seek guidance and solace from their physicians as they struggled to navigate their mortality. I had decided to change my own life's course from philosophy to medicine for the same reason. Once I completed medical school and residency, I began to set aside additional time to spend with patients and their families and set out to reprogram myself as a young physician. I started to appreciate once again the details of people's lives. Very few professions have such ready access to the contours of human life. Attentive listening — part of what it means to be a good doctor — can be therapeutic for both family and physician.

"When did you notice that Nonna was

getting sick?"

"Mama forgot the tomatoes," responded Nonna's younger son, Antonino, who then began to sob.

"Tomatoes?" I was confused.

Annunziata quickly jumped in to explain. "Five years ago, during the annual festival for Saint Anthony, Mama forgot the tomatoes for her pasta e fagioli. I came to the restaurant to help with preparations. Mama looked fine, but the stew did not. I said 'Mama, what's this? What happened to the pasta e fagioli?' She looked frightened, and then began to cry. I knew something was wrong. We went straight to the doctor. A month later, she was diagnosed with Alzheimer's. First the pasta e fagioli, then the wrong ingredients for her *ditalini* — which most of the neighborhood kids grew up on — then confusing the grandchildren with the great-grandchildren, then the night walks, the nursing home, then the fall, and now she does not eat. How can she get better without eating? This is unfair. How could this happen to someone so good, so kind?"

Healthy families are all alike; every unhealthy family is unhealthy in its own way. In their experience of illness, families are like Tolstoy's unhappy families: No two are alike. Although each patient with advanced Alzheimer's disease has similar symptoms, the ravaging of each patient's family is uniquely painful.

Once Nonna was no longer at the helm of the ship that was her family, various crew members competed to be captain. Annunziata and Antonino vied to fill Nonna's shoes. Nonna's older son was not a contender; he himself was already in the fog of the early stages of Alzheimer's disease. His three children, however, struggled for their rightful inheritance of Nonna's empire. Long-standing jealousies and simmering sibling rivalries had slowly poisoned the family dynamic. And in the midst of this family crisis, the additional burden of decision-making — when they were wholly unprepared for it — exacerbated the turmoil.

"Did you ever talk with Nonna about what sort of medical care she would want when her illness reached the advanced stages?" I asked.

Silence. And then more silence.

"Perhaps she mentioned her preferences after the death of a friend or relative? Maybe she completed a document spelling out the sort of medical care she would want?"

"Mama filled out one of those forms,"

answered Annunziata, referring to what I understood to be a health care proxy form. "After my father died in his sleep a few years ago, she named me as the person to make decisions for her when she could no longer do so."

"Did you ever talk with Nonna about what she would want if she couldn't cook anymore?"

"Mama loves life. She wants to be here with her family," Annunziata was quick to answer. "We are good Catholics. We want to be together. Do everything." She made her case in short order, and the children and grandchildren nodded in agreement. It was clear, Annunziata would be the decision-maker as Nonna traveled on her own personal Via Dolorosa.

The initial meeting is often difficult, as both parties — the family members and the physician — are feeling one another out. The family assesses if the physician is trustworthy, and the physician gauges whether the family has reasonable expectations of what medical technology can achieve. My default strategy during these early discussions is to focus on smaller discrete questions and then gradually broach broader questions. "Nonna has an infection. We are giving her antibiotics for the infection, but we need to decide whether or not to put back the feeding tube that she pulled out. Is that something you have thought about?"

"Mama needs to eat! Of course put back the feeding tube. What kind of question is that? Would you not feed your mama?" Annunziata's umbrage was palpable.

"I understand where you are coming from. We express our love for people by nourishing them. But Nonna will not get better with the feeding tube and she won't suffer without it. She has a terminal illness; the feeding tube will not make her Alzheimer's disease any better." The family gasped collectively.

I believe it is crucial to be forthright and honest with my patients and their families. Too many of my colleagues have mastered the art of verbal subterfuge and obfuscation for fear of squelching hope or in order to avoid difficult discussions, but withholding information from patients and their families prevents them from making informed decisions.

For patients with a good overall prognosis — for example, those who are unable to swallow due to neurological and neuromuscular disorders or stroke, or for patients who have had surgery on the mouth or esophagus — the feeding tube is a temporary measure to provide nutrition and give them the strength they need to survive and to get better. In patients with advanced dementia, however, the story is very different.

Medical evidence suggests that feeding tubes do not prolong survival in those patients. In 1997, a group of geriatricians from Harvard Medical School studied more than 1,300 nursing home residents with severe dementia. There was no survival benefit for residents who received a feeding tube compared to those who were not tube fed. Two years later, in 1999, a group of geriatricians from the Johns Hopkins School of Medicine pooled data from multiple studies and published similar findings in the *Journal of the American Medical Association.* In the last decade, numerous studies have found that feeding tubes in people with dementia do not prevent food from going down the wrong way (aspiration) or increase the patient's strength and weight.

But no amount of medical evidence would change Annunziata's mind. Why should it? Dr. Muriel Gillick, a nationally recognized expert in geriatrics and the use of feeding tubes, has written eloquently on this topic. "Physicians typically argue that medical interventions should have measurable medical benefit. If feeding tubes do not prolong survival, then doctors should not use them. But families focus on caring for their loved one and expressing their love. If a carefully conducted study definitively demonstrated that hugging has no effect on the immune system, no daughter would stop hugging her mother with advanced dementia. Some families feel that providing nutrition is an essential element of caring, even if it can only be administered artificially, via a feeding tube." Although I was focused on the medical evidence of feeding tubes, Nonna's daughter had other concerns on her mind.

For Annunziata, there was no greater way to express her love for her mother than to provide her with nourishment. "Mama will get better. She will get stronger, and we will get her back to the nursing home. Please put back the feeding tube, doctor." Annunziata crossed herself and the rest of her flock followed and began to pray. I am not Catholic, but I, too, bowed my head.

As the others prayed, I wondered what Nonna would have wanted had someone described to her the advanced stages of Alzheimer's disease, the devastation that her family was witnessing, the gradual annihilation of her body.

Nonna's weeping retinue dutifully filed out of the conference room and said good night. Over the next three weeks, with every passing complication, I would watch the same scene replay with the full complement of forty family members. The feeding tube was reinserted, but the infection worsened and quickly spread to Nonna's blood. Nonna was transferred back and forth between the ICU and the regular part of the hospital. What should have been a brief stay in the hospital turned into a long ordeal of mounting medical complications.

During her final transfer to the ICU, she had another tube placed down her throat to help her breathe. I visited Nonna daily, greeting her family who had camped out in the ICU's lounge to take turns sitting by her bedside. I never met a more devoted family, and I felt certain that with each ensuing deliberation they truly felt they were making the best decision for her. But with each visit I made to Nonna's bedside came an additional tube or wire chaining her to an IV bag or buzzing machine. And with each added medical intervention, my thoughts of her pain and suffering became more intense, not to mention my awareness of the wrenching torment in the eyes of her family.

My trips to visit Nonna became more frequent during the third week in the hospital. Her kidneys had begun to fail from the low blood flow to these vital organs and preparation was under way to begin dialysis. Despite the powerful medications to maintain her blood pressure, the infection was overwhelming her. On the last day of that third week, Nonna's blood pressure kept falling until it was gone. Her family was called to the bedside.

"*Basta*. Enough. Forgive us, Mama." Annunziata had made her decision for Nonna. Under her direction the entire family chanted a prayer for forgiveness. Assunta Antonia Bruno — Nonna — had died.

The images of Nonna in the ICU were seared in my mind. Worse yet, her family, from Annunziata down to the youngest great-grandchild, would have the same memories.

Nonna's last miserable weeks were as corrosive to the health of her family as dementia had been to her own life. Alzheimer's disease may have invaded Nonna's body, but the experience of her illness devastated all those around her. Could a better medical system have prevented this? Could I have prevented this?

A modest but rapidly expanding body of literature suggests that turmoil during a patient's final chapter has serious health consequences for his or her family weeks and even months after the patient's death. In 2010, the *British Medical Journal* published an article that followed families of seriously ill patients. A group of physicians who specialized in communication studied family members of patients who were admitted to a hospital and encouraged to have discussions about their values, beliefs, and goals regarding medical care. The physicians found that family members of these patients were less likely to experience stress, anxiety, and depression after the death of their loved one compared to families of patients who were not encouraged to discuss medical care. Making advance decisions about the end of life is good for a patient's health and for the health of his or her family. Doctors are unable to halt the inexorable march of Alzheimer's disease, but by encouraging these conversations early in the course of the illness, they can minimize the ravaging toll of the disease on families.

Nonna had designated a family member to assist in decision-making when she was no longer able to speak for herself. Depending on the state in which the patient lives, that individual is called a "health care proxy," "health care surrogate," "durable power of attorney for health care," "agent," or something similar. This person speaks on a patient's behalf about health decisions, including the overall goals of care. For those patients who fail to appoint a health care proxy, the process may be slower and decisions may be made by the legal next of kin or a group of people, including clinicians and family members. In rare cases, a guardian may be assigned by the court when an incapacitated patient has no health care surrogate or next of kin. Guardianship may also be needed if there are several first-degree relatives who cannot agree on treatment decisions or if it is apparent that the next of kin is not acting in the best interest of the patient.

By creating this advance directive and putting Annunziata in charge, Nonna prevented her family members from fighting for different care goals. Annunziata, and Annunziata alone, was responsible for making the decisions. Unfortunately, they never discussed what Nonna would have wanted in the event she could not cook or engage in the lives of her children and grandchildren. Nonna and Annunziata signed the paperwork without discussing the values and priorities Nonna would have wanted her daughter to consider when making medical decisions.

Without guidance from the patient, proxies are burdened with uncertainty. Simply naming a health care proxy is not enough, because proxies are not always good at predicting their loved one's wishes for medical care. In 2006, researchers at the National Institutes of Health published one of the largest studies to look at the accuracy of health care proxy decisions. They reviewed sixteen previous trials involving nearly three thousand proxy-patient pairs and discovered that health care proxies predicted patients' treatment choices with 68 percent accuracy. In other words, the probability that a daughter tells a doctor what her mom would have wanted is only somewhat better than chance. Interestingly, the researchers noted that prior discussion of preferences did not improve accuracy, although the quality of those discussions was not assessed. That being said, using informed surrogates is still the best current approach in the event that patients are unable to speak for themselves.

Patients who are planning for their own future care should consider four questions when choosing a potential health care proxy:

1. Does your proxy understand what your values and priorities are? Do you trust your proxy with your life?

2. Will your proxy be able to separate his or her feelings from yours and act on your wishes?
3. Will your proxy be a strong advocate of your expressed choices even if others — including your family members — disagree?
4. Does your proxy live near you and will he or she be available when you need help the most?

Naming a family member as a proxy can be the right choice, but not always. A close friend who knows a patient well and lives in the same city may be a better choice than a son or daughter who lives on the other side of the country and visits only every few years. When you approach someone to be your proxy, your planning is not done; in fact, it's just beginning. You and your proxy should review your directives periodically, since preferences sometimes change over time, especially over the course of a serious illness.

Patients with Alzheimer's disease need to have discussions with their proxies as early as possible in the course of the illness, when they are still able to express their wishes. The natural trajectory of Alzheimer's disease includes losing the ability to make decisions. A patient's preferences for medical care when they are in the early to middle stages of the disease, when they are still able to communicate with their loved ones and live independently, may vary greatly from their choices when they are no longer able to talk with their grandchildren or eat without assistance, but by that point they cannot make those preferences known.

Patients in the early stages of dementia must reflect on what their medical preferences would be if they were unable to do the activities that give their lives meaning and joy. To be sure, these are difficult choices, and doctors and proxies should ask patients questions like these: "What should the goals of care be when you are no longer able to speak with your loved ones? When you are no longer able to feed or bathe yourself? Should our focus be prolonging your life, providing comfort, or something in between?" Proxies wish to honor and respect patients' choices at all life stages, but they must receive guidance from the patient while he or she is still able to express these preferences.

In addition to designating and preparing a proxy, all patients should complete an additional advance directive generally known as a living will. Depending on the state in which the patient resides, it may be a standard form. Some people may feel that their wishes cannot be satisfactorily expressed by a standard form and may opt to seek legal assistance. A living will provides general insight about the patient's values and priorities, including instructions regarding what medical measures should be taken and under what circumstances. Living wills are legal documents; they are not medical orders.

Living wills should not be confused with POLST (Physician Orders for Life-Sustaining Treatment) or MOLST (Medical Orders for Life-Sustaining Treatment) forms. These forms, which are recognized in many, but not all, states, are used only for seriously ill or frail patients, and are medical orders. Living wills should also not be mistaken for DNR (Do Not Resuscitate) or the increasingly used DNAR (Do Not Attempt Resuscitation), which are orders that tell health care providers that CPR should not be performed. This is an important distinction, as standing medical orders like POLST and MOLST forms and DNR/DNAR orders are portable treatment orders and travel with the patient. Advance care directives, on the other hand, only provide legal guidance and do not apply to emergency medical personnel.

A 2010 study published in the *New England Journal of Medicine* by researchers at the University of Michigan supports the use of living wills. They studied nearly four thousand deceased adults over age sixty and found that if a patient completed a living will, that patient was less likely to want aggressive life-prolonging interventions and more likely to be cared for in a manner consistent with his or her wishes compared to patients without a living will.

Although living wills were developed as a way to help people retain control of their medical care, in reality they have not met their promise. Only about a third of American adults have an advance directive, although rates are higher among seniors. Even if a patient does complete a living will, there are still many barriers to their use. Living wills are not always readily available to doctors when they need to review the forms; they can be too vague ("If I am close to death . . .") or too specific ("If I am in a permanent coma . . .") and can be open to subjective interpretation; and they frequently need to be revisited over time as a patient's health status changes. To surmount some of these challenges, I often encourage patients to use their mobile device or tablet to memorialize their wishes on a video, and to e-mail it to their proxy and family members. In the future, patients will be able to embed such videos in their medical records so that proxies and doctors will always have access to them. Seeing a patient detailing his or her wishes is much more informative and immediate for both doctors and families than a written document.

A living will cannot anticipate every possible circumstance in which a complex medical decision may need to be made. It is practically impossible to detail wishes regarding every conceivable illness or injury that one might have in the future, and many living wills do not address situations that are related to common illnesses such as a stroke or dementia. A living will is a general guide for the medical team, and not a medical order. It is the informed health care proxy who can ensure that wishes are being honored; this is why having a knowledgeable health care proxy along with a living will is so critical.

The majority of patients admitted to hospitals today are cared for by hospitalists like me. Most patients will have never met their hospitalist prior to coming to the hospital. The same is true for my patients; I had never met Nonna or Taras prior to their admission. And although I did my very best to review their medical records and to learn as much as I could about them, they were essentially strangers to me. I did not have the opportunity to ask Nonna or Taras how they would like to live out the end of their days.

In addition to a health care proxy and a living will, all patients need to have The Conversation with their doctors, before they are too ill to do so. Since dementia is highly prevalent in older people (some estimate that half of all people over the age of eighty-five have some form of dementia), several major medical organizations, such as the Society of General Internal Medicine, the American Geriatrics Society, and the Gerontological Society of America, have promoted guidelines suggesting that physicians should have discussions about medical care for Alzheimer's disease in all patients over the age of sixty-five irrespective of whether they have been diagnosed with the illness.

Completing an advance directive — both a health care proxy form and a living will — and having a discussion about your medical care with your family, friends, and doctors are two ways to make sure that you get the care you want when you become critically ill. Sadly, many Americans never get around to any of these and suffer the same fate as Nonna and Taras did.

CHAPTER THREE:
"WE NEVER KEPT SECRETS FROM EACH OTHER"

Nonna's dementia destroyed her capacity to think and deliberate, leaving her family alone to make medical choices on her behalf. Many other patients with an advanced illness are usually too sick or delirious to have lucid discussions, and family and friends step in to process medical information and declare preferences for their medical care. Many doctors encourage patients in the early stages of a disease to start a dialogue with their family and friends about medical care, hoping that the likely future decision-makers will be well prepared to make such decisions. But a patient's willingness to discuss medical care at the end of life with his or her family and friends is not guaranteed, even among the tightest of social networks. In fact, sometimes families avoid the issue entirely, as the family of Miguel Sánchez did.

■ ■ ■ ■

"Hello, Mr. Sánchez."

"Hola . . . Doctor . . . Ángelo . . ." He slowly paused after each word, breathing in more air to gradually say the subsequent syllable. I attempted to readjust his nasal cannula, as the two pinholes delivering oxygen into his nares were plugged into his left cheek.

"¿Cómo se siente hoy?" I always made sure to address my Latino patients using the third person, a more formal greeting than the usual "¿Qué pasa?" that I would banter with my Latino colleagues. My high school Spanish teacher always reminded students to use the third person when addressing the elderly, even though most of my patients insisted I call them by their first name.

"Malo . . ." Bad. Really bad. This was probably the worst I had seen him in the three times that I had admitted him to the hospital that year alone.

Miguel Sánchez was one of my favorite patients, and also one of my frequent fliers — a patient who would return often to the hospital. In his case, the provoking event would usually be some dietary indiscretion

86

that had exacerbated his heart failure.

Heart failure is a condition that occurs when the heart cannot pump or fill with enough blood to circulate around the body. This forces the heart to work harder in order to nourish the entire body with blood. Anything that damages the heart muscle causes it to pump blood less efficiently around the body, leading to heart failure. The most common causes include high blood pressure, coronary heart disease, smoking, obesity, diabetes, and aging. Miguel, a seventy-seven-year-old obese smoker with poorly controlled diabetes, had most of the risk factors.

In one of the great ironies of the success of modern medicine, the number of patients with heart failure has skyrocketed over the last few decades due to the success of prolonging the lives of patients with heart disease and the general aging of the population. The American Heart Association estimates that there are more than five million people in the United States with heart failure.

The phrase *heart failure* is somewhat deceiving. The heart has not completely failed; it's just not as efficient as it could be. Most people do relatively well with their disease by carefully monitoring how much they exert themselves and what they eat, until something throws their system off-kilter.

Mr. Sánchez lived in a single-level ranch house with his wife in a Boston suburb. With no stairs to climb and little to do other than watch soccer games on Spanish-language television and occasionally speak to his daughter in Puerto Rico by telephone, he managed to dress and bathe himself slowly and even finish some of the light housework. His wife, Claudia, meticulously measured all the sodium content in her elaborate meals, replacing Miguel's Puerto Rican staples like chorizo (pork sausage) and *chicharrón* (fried pork rinds) with less flavorful but healthier tofu substitutes, while avoiding all canned and packaged foods. "No flavor . . ." he would grumble. Claudia persisted; she even diligently measured all the fluids that he drank, making sure he never consumed more than a liter of fluid per day.

And every now and then when his wife headed out to run errands, Miguel would surreptitiously order takeout from the local Chinese restaurant or pizzeria. One small indiscretion would disrupt the tenuous balancing act that his heart managed, pumping just enough blood with the right amount of salt and liquid throughout his body. A nugget of General Tso's chicken or a slice of pepperoni would wreak havoc with his body's steady state and bring forth all the telltale signs and symptoms of an exacerbation of heart failure: shortness of breath caused by fluid in his lungs, leg swelling, and weakness from all the added salt and fluids, along with dizziness and light-headedness.

"What was it this time, Mr. Sánchez, fried rice or pizza?"

He sat in the hospital bed simpering, but increasingly too tired from sucking in air to say anything. He was using his neck muscles to increase the force with which he could inspire more air; his chest muscles were becoming fatigued and not able to keep up with the rapid pace. When I had admitted him to the hospital in the past, he usually had been able to speak in half sentences, but this time he was worse; he could barely manage single words. He looked me straight in the eyes, and that was all I needed to see. Miguel was about to get into trouble.

The team would need to move fast. I quickly listened to his lungs with my stethoscope and then rapidly paged the respiratory therapist and nurses to assist me. "Let's get another eighty milligrams of IV Lasix to get rid of the fluid halfway up his lungs. Let's crank his oxygen to one hundred percent and change his nasal cannula to a non-rebreather. Get the noninvasive positive pressure ventilation ready if we need to use it." I quickly moved toward the head of the bed, leaning over to his ear. "Mr. Sánchez, remember what you told me the last time you were here? Did you talk with your wife and daughter about what you told me?"

"No . . . Doctor . . ." He was tired and falling asleep.

"Okay, okay. Just relax. We are here to help you," I tried to reassure him. I left the room and headed to the nurse's station. I called Claudia and asked her to come to the hospital immediately.

Heart failure is the leading cause of hospitalization in people over sixty-five years of age. More than one million Americans are hospitalized primarily for this disease each year. And for most patients with this illness, worsening of their disease is as sudden and abrupt as it was for Miguel. Just a teaspoon of salt can push someone over the edge, forcing the heart to lose its equilibrium and no longer pump enough blood to satisfy an increasingly hungry body's need for nourishing oxygen. Like a runner falling behind on a treadmill, the heart can no longer maintain the pace. The flow of blood and fluid starts to back up and flood the lungs, suffocating the patient, which is why coughing and shortness of breath are the most common symptoms.

For a sliver of heart failure patients, heart transplantation and other mechanical devices can help treat — and even cure — heart failure. But for the lion's share of people, such options are not available: The number of hearts available each year for transplants are few, and many people are too sick for mechanical devices. For most, heart failure transforms into a mercurial chronic illness characterized by repeated bouts of exacerbations interspersed with periods of relative normalcy. Miguel was like the hundreds of thousands of patients whose hearts were failing. His lungs were brimming with fluid, and we were doing our best with medicines to drain the fluid and supplement his body with oxygen. Soon, even those "Band-Aids" would not be able to keep up with him; his lungs would be drowned in fluid. It was time to have a conversation with Claudia.

"Doctor, what happened to Miguel? When I left him in the emergency room he was fine with the oxygen in his nose. But now he is not awake." Claudia was distressed.

"Mrs. Sánchez, remember when your husband was admitted to the hospital last time with fluid in his lungs?"

"Yes . . . you put the tube in his throat and put him on the breathing machine. He was in the ICU for two weeks."

"And then the rehabilitation center, and then eventually home."

"Yes."

"I'm afraid we will be at that point again soon. The medicines can only do so much. He's getting very tired of breathing."

"Not again." She struggled to remain composed, but her tears flowed copiously.

"Mrs. Sánchez, how was your husband these last few months? Was he doing the things he enjoyed, things that gave him happiness?"

"Not really. He was struggling."

"Did you speak with your husband about his wishes for medical care since the last time he was here in the hospital, maybe talk about what he would want if he ate too much salt again?"

"No. But I don't think he was happy with that tube." She pointed to her mouth.

"Did he complete any documents about

what he would want if he became really sick?"

"No."

I felt defeated.

During Miguel's last hospitalization a few months earlier, he had been intubated and placed on a breathing machine. The medicines and other measures we had taken were not sufficient, and, with his permission, we had placed a tube down his throat and connected him to a ventilator. It had been a long road to recovery; his age, obesity, smoking history, and diabetes had made "coming off" the breathing machine challenging. By the time he was able to breathe on his own, the rest of his body had started falling apart: His body's muscles had wasted away as he remained helpless on the bed for days, eventually requiring weeks of aggressive rehabilitation.

"Don't ever do that to me again!" He had not minced words with me when I visited him in the ICU after the breathing tube had eventually been removed. "That was hell," he had added in a hoarse voice.

"Sorry, Mr. Sánchez . . ." He had been transferred out of the ICU and, after some time in the regular part of the hospital, had been moved to a rehabilitation facility.

"Claudia, he told me he never wanted the tube again."

"We never really spoke about this." She was flustered.

"My impression was that he felt pretty strongly about this," I continued.

"We never kept secrets from each other . . ." She started to weep again.

"We have known each other for close to fifty years."

They had spent thousands of nights over the course of a life-time sleeping by each other's side, sharing life's most intimate secrets coupled with more mundane discussions about the weather or the next day's dinner — but not a brief exchange to inform each other about medical care at the end of life. It was at that moment that I became conscious of the fact that I, too, had not discussed my preferences for medical care with my own family. It is easy to avoid such conversations when you are feeling well and in the midst of robust health.

Claudia went on to explain how difficult the rehabilitation process had been for Miguel, including two hours of strenuous exercises each morning to strengthen his diaphragm and breathing muscles that had withered over the days on the breathing machine, followed by another two hours in the afternoon to build up his leg muscles that had wasted away. She mentioned how he had incessantly complained that the rehabilitation center had no Spanish-language television channels, and how much he missed watching his soccer games. The bland institutional food had been so unpalatable that Miguel would devour the tofu that his wife would bring on her daily visits to the center. She was not sure he would be able to go through that again and, perhaps more important, that he would want to.

"I don't think he would like that tube again, but I need to talk to our daughter, Maria. Can I call our daughter in Puerto Rico?"

"Of course."

I left the family waiting area and proceeded back to Miguel's room. He looked worse than before, his lips tinged blue and his breathing more rapid. I asked the respiratory therapist to start the noninvasive positive pressure ventilation, a type of breathing machine that connects to a patient's mouth without a tube and forces air into the lungs. It was the final measure we could offer a patient in respiratory distress before having to place a breathing tube and ventilator, unless of course a patient preferred not to be intubated.

"My daughter would like everything done. She is coming tomorrow on the next flight from Puerto Rico."

I was surprised by her statement. "Are you sure that is what your husband would want?"

"He would want to see his only daughter. He has not seen her in years."

"I understand, but do you think he would want to go through all this again?"

"Miguel loves his daughter and would want for her to be here." Claudia made her way to Miguel's side and held his hand, telling him that Maria would soon be there with them.

Miguel's breathing became more rapid and the oxygen level in his blood was falling. There was little time to wait. The noninvasive positive pressure ventilation was not sufficient. We would have to intubate him. I asked the respiratory therapist to page the anesthesiologist, who would then place a tube in Miguel's throat and connect him to a breathing machine. As the team readied for intubation, all I could hear inside my head was Miguel's voice urging me, "Don't ever do that to me again!"

Should the team have proceeded with the intubation? Miguel told me firsthand in the ICU during his previous hospitalization that he did not want to be intubated again. But was this a rash statement made in the wake of being paralyzed and stuck on a tube for a couple of weeks? Did he change his mind after the experience of successful rehabilitation and returning home to watch his soccer games and sneak in some more fried rice or pizza? When he found himself back in his home, did he regret having told me that he never wanted to be intubated? Did he decide that maybe the suffering was worth it in the end? I will never know the answers to these questions.

Claudia had felt that Miguel had been struggling and tired. His quality of life had diminished with each passing day without a soccer game or the comforts of his home. But they had never discussed his wishes should he become critically ill, despite the fact that he had been recently hospitalized. In the end, it was their daughter, Maria, who decided to pursue all life-prolonging interventions, including intubation and breathing machines. Had Miguel discussed his choices with her, perhaps on one of their phone calls? Or did Maria, guilt-ridden that she was not living nearby and caring for her father when he needed her most, make an emotional plea to her mother? The profound regret children experience during a parent's illness can be all-consuming, especially if they have been delinquent with their filial obligations. Was she making amends by pursuing all life-prolonging interventions and taking the next flight from Puerto Rico? It was not an easy choice for anyone; I still grapple with my actions and my uncertainty. What could I have done differently? What should I have done differently? I remain troubled by my choice years after it occurred.

My decision to intubate Miguel gnawed at me for some time. In an attempt to resolve my anxiety, I consulted a senior physician who was trained in both geriatrics and palliative care. "Oh, you mean the Daughter from California Syndrome?" she quickly remarked.

"No, the daughter was from Puerto Rico."

"No, the syndrome; not the patient," she added. To my surprise, there was a named syndrome to describe patients like Miguel.

In 1991, a group of geriatricians published an article in the *Journal of the American Geriatrics Society* entitled "Decision Making in the Incompetent Elderly: 'The Daughter from California Syndrome.' " The article chronicled a commonly encountered ethical conundrum in the hospital: how to care for an elderly patient with an advanced illness who no longer is able to make decisions for him or herself, the prototypical example being an elderly patient with advanced dementia.

In these situations, the medical team and family agree that treating the patient for easily reversible diseases while avoiding anything that causes pain and suffering would be the most reasonable and appropriate course for the patient. However, a long-lost distant relative — the proverbial daughter from California — suddenly arrives at the hospital and insists that the medical team pursue all aggressive life-prolonging interventions. A combination of guilt and denial are at the core of the daughter's insistence to pursue all life-prolonging interventions, not necessarily what is best for the patient. (In California, this is known as the Daughter from New York Syndrome.) Was Maria exhibiting the Daughter from Puerto Rico Syndrome?

Over the years, I have come to realize that children (and spouses) making decisions for their loved ones out of guilt and denial is quite common. It is so frequent that I started "treating" the spouses and children of patients with an advanced illness while treating the patient. It is not sufficient to only encourage patients to have The Conversation with their loved ones. I now encourage patients' families to start the discussion with their loved ones who have a serious illness.

Could Miguel's situation have been averted if his physicians, myself included, had encouraged Claudia to ask him about his wishes for medical care during his previous ICU stay? Should I have called Maria in Puerto Rico when I first met Miguel and encouraged her to start the process of exploring her father's wishes then, while he was healthy enough to talk with her?

Preventive medicine has become the focus of the practice of medicine. Many physicians have joined their public health colleagues under the tent emblazoned with the mantra "an ounce of prevention is worth a pound of cure." Did I miss an opportunity to preempt a more complicated situation by not encouraging Miguel's family — especially his daughter living far away — to approach him about having The Conversation?

For children and spouses of patients with a serious illness, I usually offer the following suggested openers to start a dialogue:

(FOR CHILDREN OF SICK PATIENTS)
"Hey, Dad, I heard that most people think it's important to talk about how they want to be treated when they are sick, but just don't get around to it. I guess they think their family will do the right thing. But if you get sick and I have to tell docs what to do, I don't want to guess what you would want. Can we talk about this? Can I ask you some questions?"

(FOR SPOUSES OF SICK PATIENTS)
"Honey, it's hard to believe that Granny (or some other recently deceased individual) is gone. But you know, hard as it was, everything was about celebrating her life. It seemed peaceful — everyone knew what was important to her and worked to make sure things were done in her way. No argument or fights. The most important thing was talking about her choices ahead of time. Can we also talk about this for the two of us?"

Engage your loved one with a serious illness gently. Let him or her know that you are open to having the discussion. In all likelihood, your loved one has thought of approaching you about the topic but feared broaching it. Start the discussion with some simple positive questions:

1. What is a good day for you now?
2. What fills your day with joy and pleasure?
3. What are you looking forward to?
4. What is important to you at this stage of your life?

And then move on to more sensitive questions:

5. What are the beliefs and values that are most important to you?
6. If you become very sick, what kinds of things would you want me to do to make sure your wishes and choices are honored?
7. Is there anything that would be helpful for me to know about how our family views serious illness?
8. Are there any cultural beliefs, practices, or preferences that we want to remember to honor?

Gauge your loved one's reaction: He or she may become tired from the emotional drain or simply from physical exhaustion. You don't have to cover every topic in one discussion. Letting him or her know that you are open to having The Conversation is the most important signal that you can give.

And when the discussion ends, remember always to be appreciative and to say "I love you."

When patients have a serious illness like the advanced stages of heart failure, cancer, or dementia, the decisions that need to be made in the future are foreseeable. Whether or not to have CPR, a breathing machine, or a feeding tube are predictable decision points that will arise as the disease progresses. Had Claudia or Maria started this discussion earlier with Miguel, they would never have been left to guess — or worse, insist — on medical care for him. Unfortunately, it was already too late to have an exchange with Miguel. He was unable to speak now due to a tube in his throat and high doses of sedating medications.

The following afternoon, I decided to visit Miguel in the ICU. He was no longer on my medical service; the ICU doctors were in charge of his medical care. But it was always difficult to let go of a patient who weighed heavily on my conscience.

Miguel looked comfortable despite having a tube down his throat. His lips were back to their normal pink color, and he breathed at a leisurely fourteen breaths per minute. He was heavily sedated and unable to speak with me. I went to the family lounge looking for Claudia, and perhaps their daughter Maria.

"Doctor, this is my daughter Maria."

"Hello, Doctor. Thank you for taking such good care of my father."

"Your dad is very special, as I am sure you know . . . Unfortunately he can't stay away from the Chinese food and pizza." We all laughed.

"Can I ask you something?" Maria nodded. "Had you spoken with your father about his wishes for medical care, about whether he would want to be in the ICU again?"

"No, we didn't. I haven't spoken to him in months. With the kids and work and his illness, you know . . . It's tough being so far away . . . But it's good to be here now with my parents to support them and get him home."

Home? Did she really think that Miguel was going home this time? Despite aggressive use of powerful medicines to remove the fluid from Miguel's lungs and strengthen his heart, the ICU doctors had been unable to remove him from the ventilator. He also started to suffer the many complications that older, obese, diabetic patients get in the hospital: infections, muscle wasting, and delirium.

After Miguel had been connected to the ventilator for two weeks, doctors created a hole in his trachea so that the tube in his mouth could be removed and placed directly through his throat. Claudia and Maria agreed to the tracheostomy and also gave consent to have a feeding tube placed so that nutrition could be continued. He was eventually transferred to a nursing home, where he would likely remain dependent on a ventilator for breathing and a feeding tube for fluids and electrolytes. Throughout all this, Miguel was either heavily sedated or too delirious to communicate with his family or staff. Decisions were being made on his behalf even though he had no say in the matter.

I never found out what happened to Miguel. I would be surprised if he ever was able to breathe on his own again, watch a soccer game, or taste General Tso's chicken. His obesity, smoking history, diabetes, and advanced heart failure had taken their toll on his body.

If he ever did wake up from his delirium,

I feared how he would interrogate me. "Dr. Ángelo, did you not hear me when I said to never let them do this to me?" How would I respond?

"But your daughter insisted . . ."

I frequently imagine how my patients with advanced illnesses would cross-examine me regarding their medical care. "Dr. Ángelo, based on what evidence did you proceed with my intubation? Didn't you have reason to believe that I would prefer not to have been intubated?"

Or perhaps less charitably, "Dr. Ángelo, you took an oath to first do no harm and yet you allowed a hole to be placed in my throat that would never allow me to talk again and a hose in my stomach forbidding me to ever experience the joy of tasting food. How do you justify your actions? Would you do this to your father?"

How would I plead? What would I say?

Had someone years ago described to my patients and their families the later stages of diseases like heart failure, dementia, and cancer and all the medical interventions that might be attempted, maybe they would have chosen differently. Maybe this all could be avoided. But sometimes words cannot accurately capture the devastation patients experience and their loved ones witness; sometimes seeing is believing.

Chapter Four:
"Where Do We Go from Here?"

On the first Friday in September at precisely eight A.M., Professor Helen Thompson prepared to deliver arguably the greatest lines of American poetry. She was about to embark on a semester-long journey exploring American poetry. Exposing young minds to words that moved generations was her singular mission in life.

> I celebrate myself, and sing myself,
> And what I assume you shall assume,
> For every atom belonging to me as good
>   belongs to you.

She never read from notes, and she performed with the level of aplomb that only the most senior professors seem to possess. Her course on Whitman, Dickinson, Frost, Stevens, Williams, Crane, Bishop, Roethke, and Ammons attracted only the brightest and most serious students. What other college-aged students would attend a poetry class at the ungodly hour of eight A.M.? She was not about to waste her time reading poetry with just anyone. "I want students with soul. Students who could become my *Leaves of Grass.*"

I loafe and invite my soul,
I lean and loafe at my ease observing a
  spear of summer grass.

The professor's thirty-first time reciting Whitman's famous lines on the first day of school, however, was about to go awry.

My tongue, every atom of my blood, form'd
  from this soil, this air,
Born here of parents born here from
  parents the same, and their parents the
  same . . .

And then silence. She stared straight ahead and her students grew increasingly anxious. The silence was deafening, but after what seemed like an interminable minute, Helen continued as if nothing had happened.

I, now thirty-seven years old in perfect
  health begin,
Hoping to cease not till death.

109

When I first met Helen nine months later, she did not remember this event. She was no longer the assured professor who delivered poems as performance pieces to teach and inspire. When I admitted her to the hospital, Helen was fifty-six years old and had been diagnosed with aggressive glioblastoma multiforme; a six-centimeter brain tumor was crushing her brain. An expanding butterfly-shaped growth had extinguished a lifetime's worth of verse in less than a year.

As I found out later from her primary care doctor at the university, she had visited the health clinic three times that year. During the first visit, right after her lapse in the classroom, she was told that she was likely working too hard — a reasonable diagnosis given her style and personality — and that she should ease her jam-packed schedule. At the second visit, she was given some muscle relaxants and told to return if the symptoms persisted, advice that eluded her failing memory. On the third visit, her primary care doctor ordered a CT scan that discovered the brain lesion.

A neurosurgeon immediately performed a biopsy of the mass. The diagnosis was unequivocal: glioblastoma multiforme. Most cancers are lethal, but some kill you faster than others. Glioblastoma is one of the swiftest.

The number of cells comprising the brain is unparalleled. In addition to the billions of nerve cells called neurons that transmit electrical impulses and form synapses, half of the volume of the brain consists of quadrillions of glial cells. Glial cells are the glue of the brain (*glia* is Greek for "glue"), performing housekeeping functions by nourishing and repairing neurons and perhaps so much more. Unfortunately for thousands of patients each year, glial cells are also the source of nearly all forms of brain cancer.

In many ways, the body is like real estate; what matters most is location, location, location. In the body, there is no location more valuable, exclusive, or limited than the brain, which is why the brain is enclosed in a Fort Knox–worthy shell, the skull. Any brain cancer is inherently serious and life-threatening because of the scarce room available. Unlike Manhattan real estate, where building ever-higher skyscrapers is always an option, in the skull there are very few places to go except for down, and a growing tumor can begin to squeeze the base of the brain and the spinal cord while increasing the pressure in the skull.

Glioblastoma multiforme grows very, very fast. By the time you have symptoms, the tumor has already spread its tentacles into the brain, and consequently, these tumors can rarely be surgically removed. In Helen's case, the tumor had started on one side of the brain, in the frontal lobe, but was increasing at an alarming pace. It had already crossed over to the other side of her brain, giving the tumor a butterfly appearance.

On the day I met her, Helen had complained to colleagues that her headaches were worsening. When she had started vomiting, she was rushed by ambulance to the emergency room. Her brain was literally being crushed by the pressure, and her immediate survival was in danger.

"Let's get some dexamethasone and mannitol immediately," I said to one of the nurses. It was the beginning of my shift and I was the overnight doctor on duty. "Let's get the patient hooked up to a heart monitor. Betty, did we administer another dose of dexamethasone and mannitol? . . . Todd, please bring up the films from the emergency department on the laptop. And someone call the next of kin." The nurses were accustomed to this barrage of commands and responded immediately. Treating tumors in the skull was an oft-practiced page from the cancer playbook, and everybody worked together in a well-trained team.

The glioblastoma multiforme had its own strategy, however, and Helen was becoming slightly less responsive. Still, her occasional grimace at the poke or prod of a needle reminded all of us that she was conscious of what we were doing. But time was not on our side. By now she was capable of responding only to loud stimuli, which startled her. She received the first few doses of the appropriate medications in the emergency room; now we had to wait.

When I reviewed the films from the emergency department, I could not help wondering how something so beautiful could be so lethal.

Helen's tumor was causing inflammation and swelling in her brain, and this was disrupting the precise neuronal synapses that had allowed her to effortlessly recite long passages from Whitman. The steroid dexamethasone was given to decrease the inflammation and mannitol, a diuretic, was prescribed to decrease the swelling.

In patients with nonterminal brain cancers, a neurosurgeon can perform a craniotomy, in which part of the skull is temporarily removed to relieve some of the

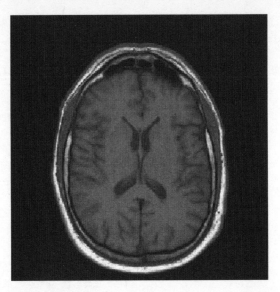

Normal Brain MRI Image: This bird's-eye view from above is called the sagittal view.

pressure on the brain. But Helen's glioblastoma multiforme, or butterfly glioma for short, was terminal. The tumor was inoperable, and in the previous months her doctors had attempted to decrease its size with radiation and chemotherapy, but to no avail. At best, the medicines we were giving her would only temporarily relieve some of the pressure; and a craniotomy would make no difference in the end.

"Okay," I continued, "be aggressive with the medications. They'll kick in soon enough, over the next few hours. I want you to check her neurological status every half

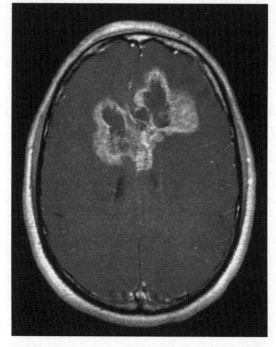

Butterfly Glioma MRI (Sagittal View)

hour. Page me if there is any change or if her family arrives." I was already getting called back to the emergency department for my next admission.

Within a few hours, the nurses paged me to reevaluate Helen; her husband, Charles, had arrived by then. When I walked into her room, the two were tightly clasping hands.

Once I introduced myself to Helen and Charles, I gave them both an update. The dexamethasone and mannitol had kicked in

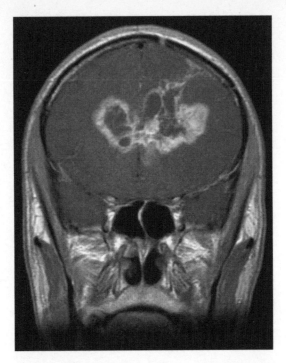

Butterfly Glioma (Coronal View): Imagine that the brain has been split from front to back between the ears. This is the frontal view.

and Helen's intracranial pressure was no longer an immediate threat to her life. But for how long?

"How are you feeling?" I asked her.

"Looks like I had quite an eventful day, but I'm none the worse for wear. When can I get back to my class and students?"

Back to her class and students? Was she still teaching? Did she understand the terminal nature of her disease? Hadn't her

primary care doctor, oncologist, or neurosurgeon talked with her about the likely
course of her disease?

In many cases, within minutes after meeting, hospitalized patients and doctors must
discuss life-and-death decisions. They're in
the hospital for urgent care, and, more often
than not, their regular doctors have not
previously broached the issue of end-of-life
care. It is a travesty and a disservice. I
always ask my patients' outpatient doctors
if they had started a conversation with the
patient about end-of-life care. Almost
inevitably they say no and give some version of the following response: "I didn't get
around to it yet. I was hoping to talk about
it at the next visit." But who am I to blame
them? Primary care doctors have, on average, about fourteen minutes per patient
visit. Is it conceivable to address end-of-life
care in so little time?

The absolute worst time to contemplate
decisions about medical care is when one is
critically ill and in the hospital. Feeling
dreadfully sick and, perhaps, vomiting or in
pain, patients are completely disoriented
amid the foreign surroundings and new
doctors. Unfortunately, this is often when a
decision must be made.

At this stage, the physician summarizes

for the patient the medical facts as he or she sees them, lists the possible interventions with their accompanying risks and benefits, and ends with the disclaimer "There is some uncertainty in everything I have just said. Medicine is still part art and part science." At the dawn of the twentieth century, William Osler, often referred to as the father of modern medicine, told a graduating class of medical students: "A distressing feature in the life of which you are about to enter . . . is the uncertainty which pertains not alone to our science and art, but to the very hopes and fears which make us men. In seeking out the absolute truth we aim for the unattainable, and must be content with finding broken portions."

It is no less true today. Although doctors have a clearer sense of the prognosis when looking at the big picture for certain illnesses, there will always be some degree of uncertainty in medicine, and it is hard to be content with finding broken portions.

"Helen, have you discussed with your other doctors the course of your illness? Perhaps you and Charles talked with your oncologist?"

"No, not particularly. We were all focused on fighting the tumor with all available treatments," she said, as Charles nodded in agreement.

"The brain tumor is getting larger rapidly," I told her. "We are trying our best to decrease some of the brain swelling with medications, but these are only temporary measures. Unfortunately, the cancer will continue to grow."

"Oh dear, that sounds rather concerning. How large has it grown?"

Her films were still on the laptop screen that the team had reviewed earlier, and with some slight hesitation I showed Helen and her husband the images.

"Clouds. My mind is filled with innumerable clouds. I never fathomed that this is what the tumor looks like. How can I think amid so much haze?" She took a deep breath and then a tear streaked down her cheek. Charles held her hand more tightly. "Where do we go from here?" she asked me.

Where do we go from here? There were two roads to take and one cannot travel both (even though the destination remains the same). And both roads are equally good — or bad. Neither could be said to be grassier or less traveled. Helen would make a decision and never know what would have happened if she had chosen differently.

My job was to give Helen and Charles the

lay of the land.

"Helen, your tumor is pushing on your brain and may cause fatal brain herniation, the squeezing of your brain out of the skull. We are trying our best to avoid this by decreasing the swelling with medicines, but they may not be enough."

I could hear myself reciting a litany of increasingly obscure terms, conditions, and treatments. "The medicines are just temporary measures," I continued. "In all likelihood, the tumor will keep growing, and then these interventions won't help."

"Is there anything else you can do if the medicines stop working?"

"Unfortunately, chemotherapy and radiation failed to shrink the tumor, and the neurosurgeon will not perform another surgery because it won't change the final outcome."

Silence.

I was trying to give Helen an accurate picture of what she could expect, but I was suffocating and began to grasp for something to add. "Well, in some patients who do not respond to the dexamethasone and mannitol and become critically ill, we can try hyperventilating the lungs to decrease the amount of carbon dioxide in the blood, which decreases swelling in the brain." I was

120

spouting anything and everything but the obvious truth: Helen had a terminal cancer and was dying.

"What's my alternative?"

"Well, we can carefully monitor you and continue to give you medicines to decrease the swelling. We can make sure that you are not in any discomfort and give you painkillers if you're uncomfortable. If we go down this road, you can spend time outside of the hospital with Charles at home."

"What happens at the end?"

"In the end, the intracranial pressure becomes untenable, causing the blood pressure to elevate drastically, the lungs to stop breathing, and the heart to slow down until it stops. It's called Cushing's Triad."

A bead of sweat ran down my forehead. Had I really just said "Cushing's Triad"? I was hiding behind medical jargon. What I really needed to say to Helen was that no matter what anyone might do, she would die very soon.

"Well, we shouldn't just sit back and not fight. I am a fighter. Do whatever you need to fix me. I have more students to teach next semester," she proclaimed, seemingly unaware that there was simply no way she could win this battle.

The idea that people can control a terminal illness if they can muster the courage to fight is probably deeply ingrained in our cultural DNA, along with the denial of death and other Promethean ambitions. No large, well-conducted, scientific study has ever shown a significant association between personality traits and survival from cancer, but my guess is that no number of negative studies will ever extinguish this deeply held belief.

We see cancer patients battling death as valiant, and we think that if they try hard enough, they'll beat it. In truth, cancer is an equal-opportunity killer and is impervious to moral virtues and emotional strength. No amount of courage increases a patient's likelihood of survival. For every courageous patient who survives, there is another courageous patient who does not. Of course you'd never know that from popular media, where patients wage battle against cancer and win, and where almost everyone survives CPR and looks remarkably good hooked up to a breathing machine.

In one oft-quoted study published in the *New England Journal of Medicine* in 1996, a group of doctors watched all the episodes from three popular medical television shows (*ER, Chicago Hope,* and *Rescue 911*) broadcast during 1994–95. They found sixty occurrences of CPR in ninety-seven television episodes reviewed. When they analyzed the success rate of CPR in these shows, 75 percent of patients on television survived CPR.

Unfortunately, cancer does not follow the usual Hollywood script. Two recent studies led by critical-care doctors and published in the journals *Critical Care* and the *New England Journal of Medicine* in 2010 and 2009, respectively, suggest that the success rate of CPR (defined as being alive at the time of hospital discharge) ranges between 8 to 18 percent, depending on the age and health of the patient. But even those percentages are deceiving. Both studies looked at all patients who had cardiac arrest — those who had an advanced illness as well as those who were very healthy. An otherwise healthy sixty-five-year-old man who recently had completed the Boston marathon and presents with sudden cardiac arrest from a blocked heart artery has an excellent chance of success with immediate resuscitation, as does the healthy eighty-year-old woman who has no chronic illnesses. CPR and resuscitation frequently do work with those types of patients; but these numbers are misleading to seriously ill patients, who have vastly different results.

For seriously ill patients, the more relevant question is: What is the success rate for CPR in patients like me, who have my stage of disease? Even though on television most people survive CPR, in real life most patients with a terminal illness do not. In one study published in 2009 in the journal *Supportive Care in Cancer,* sixty-one patients with terminal advanced cancer (patients just like Helen) and who had cardiac arrest underwent resuscitation. Of the sixty-one patients who had CPR, only ten patients (11 percent) were resuscitated successfully and regained a pulse. The average survival time for these ten patients was three hours. No patient became conscious after the cardiac arrest, and no patient left the hospital alive.

In the abstract, fighting every second of the way and pursuing aggressive life-prolonging interventions sounds admirable — but did Helen understand what this entailed? Did she appreciate the possible suffering it involved? How about the likely outcome? How could I paint a realistic portrait to help her imagine the unimaginable?

I would respect and support Helen and Charles's resolution. But I wanted to ensure that they were making a truly informed decision. "Do you mind if we go on a tour of the hospital?" I asked them.

I swaddled Helen in a blanket and placed her in a wheelchair along with her numerous IVs and heart monitor. Charles accompanied us as I wheeled her to the elevator, which we took up one floor to the ICU. I pushed Helen in the wheelchair around the unit, while Charles trailed not too far behind. It was the middle of the night and no one seemed to mind. I didn't have a set itinerary and so we meandered from room to room, enough to feel the rhythm of the place.

From a distance, Helen and Charles viewed a patient on a ventilator as well as a patient on hemodialysis. One of the physicians was performing a lumbar puncture on a feverish patient with sepsis and another was placing a central line in the neck vein of a patient with metastatic colon cancer. It was a routine evening in the ICU, but Helen and Charles scanned every square inch of the place, taking in each detail slowly and methodically.

"Code Blue, ICU! Code Blue, ICU!" A phalanx of nurses ran ahead of us toward one of the rooms down the hall. "Both of you, please stay here," I told Helen and Charles. As the overnight physician, I assisted with all the codes in the ICU. I hurried in hot pursuit of the nursing team.

One of the ICU doctors was at the foot of the patient's bed giving orders. The nurses, who had already started CPR, filled me in on some of the details of the patient: a ninety-two-year-old female with widely metastatic colon cancer. Earlier that day, the family had been deliberating about the goals of medical care for her and wondered if life-prolonging interventions in the ICU made sense given her grim prognosis. They had decided to take an additional day to sort things out. Regrettably, her disease wasn't about to wait.

I grabbed a pair of gloves to assist with chest compressions. The ICU doctor had cycled through three rounds of medications to restart the patient's heart and continued compressions. The ICU doctor barked, "Please stop compressions, and let's check for a pulse."

As I was about to switch places with one of the nurses performing CPR, I caught something out of place out of the corner of my eye — people not wearing hospital scrubs or a white coat. It was Helen and Charles. I let a nurse take my place and I escorted them both down the hall and out of the ICU.

As we made our way back to Helen's room, I apologized.

"It's okay, Angelo. You helped us more than you will ever know."

"I wanted you to understand what could happen in the ICU, but I didn't mean for the two of you to see that code."

"Please, it's all right. I wish I hadn't seen the last few minutes of the tour, but it's important that patients and families see what we're talking about. I had no idea."

"Please get some rest," I said. "I will see you both again tomorrow."

Early the next morning, as my shift was winding down, the fresh morning doctors stopped by the lounge to pick up their lists of overnight patients. Areej, a dazzling young doctor, was going to take over Helen's care. "Please make sure to keep a close eye on Professor Thompson," I told her. "She's alert now, but who knows for how long? Unfortunately, none of her doctors ever talked with her about goals of care. Last night she insisted she wanted to fight, but make sure to discuss the plan going forward with her and her husband. I'll check back in with her tonight when I return." I signed my pager over to Areej and headed home exhausted.

When I returned to the hospital that evening, I immediately went to check on Helen, but her room was empty. I scanned the marker board at the nurses' station that had all the patients listed by initials. E.A., P.V., H.B., W.K., A.D., T.C., J.V., A.T, and M.A., but no H.T. I paged Areej frantically, fearing the worst.

"She went home with hospice care," reported Areej. "After discussing the likely course of the tumor and the options, Professor Thompson decided to go home on steroids for the swelling. A visiting hospice nurse will check in on her daily in case she becomes uncomfortable and needs pain meds. A group of her students are creating a schedule for taking turns to sleep over at her home to keep an eye on her along with her husband."

I had been so overwhelmed with the medical science, citing all the arcane medical details, that I had missed the opportunity to talk about her other options, such as hospice. Doctors too often become so preoccupied with the medical facts that they lose sight of the forest for the trees.

When medical care cannot provide a cure, hospice reorients the care toward comfort. This does not mean that the health care system has given up on the patient. Rather, hospice teams include doctors, nurses, social workers, counselors, pharmacists, chaplains, and others who work to keep patients free of symptoms and pain by providing medicines, medical supplies, and physical therapy if needed, while offering both patients and families counseling and assistance with the spiritual and emotional aspects of dying.

Hospice is a benefit paid for by Medicare, Medicaid, and most private insurers. Hospice care usually is provided in the patient's home, but for some patients whose pain cannot be controlled at home or who lack adequate social support, hospice can be provided in the hospital, nursing home, or even a dedicated hospice home.

There is growing evidence that patients who choose a more comfort-oriented approach earlier in the course of their illness actually live longer. A 2007 study conducted by researchers at the National Hospice and Palliative Care Organization and published in the *Journal of Pain and Symptom Management* looked at the difference in survival periods in two groups of terminally ill Medicare patients — those who used hospice services and those who did not. On average, the mean survival period was nearly one month longer for the patients who received comfort care. It was longer for patients who had congestive heart failure (eighty-one more days), lung cancer (thirty-nine more days), pancreatic cancer (twenty-one more days), and colon cancer (thirty-three more days). Two main factors were at play. First, hospice avoided the intensive medical interventions associated with higher mortality rates; and second, hospice provided patients with interdisciplinary care coordination and medications that might not be otherwise covered. These findings were contrary to the widespread belief among many health care providers and the wider public that medicines used to relieve pain may hasten death.

Similar results were seen in a landmark 2010 study conducted by oncologists at the Massachusetts General Hospital in Boston and published in the *New England Journal of Medicine*. Lung cancer patients receiving early comfort-oriented care lived nearly 25 percent longer (nearly three months) than their counterparts who delayed such care. As the authors state, "With earlier referral to a hospice program, patients may receive care that results in better management of symptoms, leading to stabilization of their condition and prolonged survival."

Comfort care should not be equated with early death. Based on these studies, innovative new models of hospice care are being developed in which comfort care is being delivered simultaneously with standard medical care. Future work in this area will likely provide more insights into how we can better provide care to the dying.

Areej's report of Helen's decision left me speechless.

"I think you were the first person to be honest and tell them that the tumor was really bad and unlikely to change course," she said. "Both of them wanted to spend as much time at home reading poetry together, comfortable and outside of the hospital."

I could breathe again.

"They mentioned their tour of the ICU," Areej continued, "and how much it helped them understand what you were talking about. They said to say good-bye to you and to thank you. That was really cool of you to take them to the ICU. Really cool."

■ ■ ■ ■

I take care of hundreds of patients over the course of the year and don't always see how things turn out. Following the stories of so many patients after they leave the hospital is nearly impossible. Not knowing what happens to them is like starting to read a book and never reaching the final chapter, or starting a movie only to stop it right before the denouement.

But a few weeks after my conversation with Areej, I caught a headline as I read the local paper on a lazy weekend afternoon: HELEN THOMPSON, RENOWNED SCHOLAR, DIES AT 56. The obituary, written by one of her former students, was three columns long and extolled Helen's illustrious career. I, however, was much more interested in the first few lines: "Professor Helen Thompson, a renowned scholar, died yesterday at her home. She was fifty-six. The cause was brain cancer."

She had died at home, in the company of her husband and surrounded by the works of Walt Whitman. Helen had gotten her final wish.

Hospice is not for everyone. Some patients

are willing to tolerate profound pain, suffering, and inconveniences in order to eke out some more time. They choose to pursue all life-prolonging interventions in the face of grave illness. And sometimes these interventions do in fact prolong a patient's life. I learned this important lesson not long after I met Helen Thompson.

Elijah Jones was a seventy-nine-year-old descendant of share-croppers on a former slave plantation in the Deep South. When he looked in the face of his own impending death — from kidney failure, a bad heart, and other ailments — and evaluated the terrible odds of successful treatment, he chose a very different course: He wanted it all.

At the time, I was surprised at the speed with which Mr. Jones responded after hearing his options. Starting dialysis at his age was not a decision to be taken lightly. Two heart attacks and a stroke had already forced him into a nursing home. If he had been a hale and hearty seventy-nine, starting dialysis would have been the obvious choice, but he was far from the ideal of robust older health. He was chronically ill, debilitated from a stroke, unable to walk or dress himself, and constantly short of breath from a weak heart.

But he had seen much worse over the

course of a long, hard life. By his own account, Elijah should have been dead years earlier. "I've been through hell and back, son, and God has given me a second chance before He calls me home. I'll do anything to live some more. I've been through harsher things than this."

I admired his resilience.

Elijah Jones had lived through some of the most tumultuous years in this country's history. Growing up in the deeply segregated South during the early to middle part of the twentieth century was grueling. Verbal abuse and physical violence were part of the life experience for many African-Americans. Elijah said he had come to dread his long walks home from school through hostile neighborhoods, but he persisted because he and his family saw education as a ticket to a better life. Despite being first in his high school class and eventually graduating from his local college with an engineering degree, the best job he could get back then was as a short-order cook in a local luncheonette.

By the time of the civil rights movement in the 1960s, Elijah had settled down in a small home — a shack really, with no indoor plumbing. He packed off his only child, a daughter, to the Northeast in the early 1970s to seek a better education and a better life. If he could not live his dream, at least she could. He did not leave the Deep South with her, for he never expected to grow old.

Growing up, many of the funerals he attended in his Baptist church were of men fairly young by today's standards, mostly in their fifties and occasionally in their sixties. He never figured he'd make it to sixty-five and regretted paying his Social Security and Medicare taxes with each paycheck since he was sure he'd never reap the benefits. When his wife died at the age of fifty-nine from a massive stroke, he was sure he would be next.

For most of his life, Elijah was told he had high blood pressure, but he couldn't afford routine health care and the medications needed to control his hypertension. By the time he did reach sixty-five and qualified for treatment under Medicare, the damage had already been done. His heart, brain, and kidneys began to fail him. Over the next decade, he suffered two heart attacks and a stroke, leaving his heart unable to pump blood efficiently and the left side of his body weak. His daughter, now a successful professional in the Northeast, traveled back and forth to see him every few weeks, eventually moving him into a nursing home in the

South. Despite doing her best to juggle her schedule, the trips back home were becoming increasingly difficult to manage, and she ultimately relocated her father hundreds of miles north to a nursing home closer to her home.

Elijah slowly adjusted to life in the nursing home, but soon, he was not urinating as frequently. He began to leave half of his dinner tray uneaten and spent most of his time in bed. The nursing home doctor was alerted and a blood test revealed the root of his problem: His kidneys were failing. He was admitted to the hospital for further evaluations and I was the doctor in charge of figuring out what to do.

"Hi, Mr. Jones, my name is Dr. Volandes. Angelo is my first name. Sorry to interrupt lunch, but I'll be taking care of you." I moved his lunch tray to the side and pulled a chair over to chat with him.

"Yes, sir. Glad to meet you."

"Why don't you tell me about yourself? I noticed your Southern accent. I assume you're not from around here?"

Elijah proceeded to tell me about his life in the South: his wife, his daughter, the phenomenal Southern fried cooking, his longings for the warm summer evenings of his past, and the strength of his church's fellowship.

"What sort of things make you happy now?"

"I love the Lord, and I love going to church, but I can't do that anymore. I listen to my gospel music, though, and every day I live is a blessing."

"I was hoping we could talk through some of your options and then you can discuss them with your family."

"Just my daughter now. But I'll do whatever you say — you're the M.D."

I told him that his kidneys were not working as well as they should.

"There's lots of me that isn't working all that well."

"Well, if your kidneys stop cleaning your blood, you could die. I've tried looking for some causes of your kidney problems that we can fix, but it looks like you may have had this for some time. Now that your kidneys are shutting down, we need to think about what to do. I want to talk to you about . . . dialysis as well as some other options, and then together we can decide what makes sense for you."

Dialysis follows a strict routine. The usual regimen includes visiting a dialysis center three times a week for about three hours each time. During each visit, the patient is hooked with a needle to a dialysis machine through a surgically placed access site on the patient's arm called a fistula. Blood is circulated to the dialysis machine, cleaned, and then returned to the patient through another needle.

Close to four hundred thousand Americans receive dialysis and lead normal lives. I have had many patients, some older than Elijah, start dialysis and do quite well. And although for thousands of people being on dialysis results in a positive overall experience, there is increasing evidence indicating that many frail elderly nursing home residents with multiple medical issues often do poorly after starting the treatment. In one large study published in 2009 in the *New England Journal of Medicine,* nephrologists studied more than three thousand nursing home residents who were followed for twelve months after starting dialysis. By the end of one year, 58 percent had died, and 87 percent had experienced significant and sustained decline in their abilities to perform activities such as walking, bathing, getting out of bed, and using the toilet. Dialysis may prolong life for some, but it often does not preserve physical and mental functioning, leading to increasing dependence on others to assist with basic functions of life.

It is a difficult trade-off.

The mounting evidence suggesting that dialysis may not be helpful in frail older patients led to a significant change in the national guidelines for dialysis. The new guidelines recommend forgoing dialysis in patients over seventy-five who have multiple significant medical problems and who are unable to perform basic activities of daily living. In other words, for patients like Elijah.

The lead author of the guidelines was Dr. Alvin "Woody" Moss, an internationally recognized expert on decision-making regarding dialysis. I asked Woody about the committee's decision to change the guidelines regarding dialysis in patients like Elijah. "There was accumulating evidence that indicated many elderly patients started on dialysis fared badly. Whether or not to start dialysis in an elderly patient with numerous comorbidities and a poor prognosis should be a shared decision based on an informed patient's values and preferences and a physician's recommendation. Dialysis is a procedure just like any other medical intervention. The most current clinical practice guideline underlines the importance of a comprehensive informed consent process based on the best available evidence." It was time to share in the decision-making with Elijah.

After exploring what was important to him at this stage in his life, I did my best to explain the process of dialysis, the frequent visits he'd make to the dialysis center, the fistula that would need to be created surgically in his arm, the need for temporary catheters in his neck until his permanent fistula was ready for use, and the statistics about survival for patients like him. Then I told him about the alternative to dialysis.

"We can focus on making you feel as good as possible without dialysis. The attention would be on your quality of life rather than prolonging it. Doctors would continue to support you, making sure you eat a special diet and take medicines to slow down your kidney disease and manage your symptoms."

"How long I got without dialysis?"

How long would he live? This question is always one of the most difficult to answer, particularly in the context of kidney failure. Among patients whose kidneys are failing, there remains a good deal of residual kidney function. How long a patient with kidney failure lives can vary greatly; just a few weeks for some, months for others, and even more for still others. In fact, the humorist and opinion columnist Art Buchwald made skipping dialysis a cause célèbre.

At the age of eighty, Buchwald had decided to stop dialysis for his kidney failure. Tired of being tied to a dialysis clinic and having to adhere to the strict nutritional diet, Buchwald decided to live life the way he wanted, eating lots of fast food, full of sodium and potassium, with relish. He thought he would live at most a week or two, but weeks turned into months. Soon his kidneys had recovered enough that he returned to writing his humorous opinion pieces, even publishing a book on his experience. Age eventually does catch up, however. Almost one year to the date that he announced his decision to stop dialysis, he died at his son's home. Was Buchwald a statistical outlier? Could Elijah be one, too? I was filled with uncertainty.

"I am not sure, Mr. Jones. It's really difficult to predict. For some people, it can be weeks, for others months, and for some lucky few, maybe longer."

"Where do we go from here?"

"Well, it depends. It's a quality-versus-quantity issue. Do you want to focus on your quality of life or your quantity of life? If you value quality, then avoiding fistula surgery, needles, and thrice-weekly trips to a dialysis center would mean better quality, but it might mean fewer days of life. But if you're more interested in the quantity of your days, then dialysis would help clean your blood of waste products and hopefully give you a longer life. But as I mentioned, older folks who live in nursing homes and have other diseases don't always fare very well on dialysis. They often have complications like infections and blood clots."

"Could I take a look at this dialysis?"

Some dialysis centers offer tours to patients, allowing them to meet the nursing staff and have an orientation prior to receiving treatment. I called down to arrange it. I knew this tour would be less eventful than Helen's.

With some assistance, I put Elijah in a wheelchair and rolled him down to the unit. It was lunchtime, so there were no patients, giving the place something of an eerie feeling. Half of the room was filled with blue recliners with large armrests for connecting the dialysis needle. Patients could sit and relax in the chairs, which were flanked by a small television on one side and a loudly whirring dialysis machine on the other. The other half of the room had no chairs — just a row of dialysis machines. This half would soon be packed with the stretchers of patients too weak to sit in a dialysis chair for three hours. Elijah would likely be in this half of the room.

One of the dialysis nurses came over and explained to Elijah the usual routine for patients and what he could expect.

"Can I take a look at the needle?" he asked.

She brought over sterile dialysis needles that were still in their plastic casing. They were thicker than the needles most hospitals use for daily blood draws, and about an inch or so in length.

"Is that what all the fuss is about?" He clearly didn't think much of the needles.

We returned to his room. "Why don't you take some time to think about all this," I said. "There's no need for you to decide today. Maybe discuss it with your daughter, and we can talk it over again in the morning."

But he had made up his mind. "I want it all."

The following morning I met with Elijah again, this time along with his daughter. She was hesitant about the dialysis, and she certainly didn't like the odds for elderly patients like her father. If more than half of people died after a year on dialysis and most of those who were still alive had problems with daily activities, why not just focus on quality of life? We looked at each other, thinking the same thing. But she acceded to her father's wishes, and we settled on a trial of dialysis to see how things would go.

Within days, the surgeons created a fistula, but it would be a few months before it was ready for use. In the interim, large catheters were placed in Elijah's neck so he could start dialysis. For the first week, he stayed in the hospital to receive his initial treatments, and he was soon transferred back to the nursing home. Once the fistula in his arm was healed, his neck catheters were removed and the fistula was used for the treatment.

For about fourteen months, things progressed fairly well. He would listen to his gospel music while the whirring dialysis machine extracted the deadly urea from his blood. But then complications set in and the fistula became clogged with blood clots.

Elijah was admitted to the hospital. The doctors caring for him placed temporary catheters in his groin. He continued his dialysis in the hospital but soon became feverish and unresponsive. His groin catheters had become infected. He was transferred to the ICU for closer monitoring because of his tenuous blood pressure. He was started on antibiotics and numerous medications to maintain his blood pressure.

In the ICU, he was barely conscious. The nurses had placed a radio by his bedside, filling the room with gospel music, and his daughter visited in the evenings. After Elijah had been in the ICU for a few weeks, his daughter decided on his behalf that his time had come. God was calling him. Late one Saturday morning, the dialysis, antibiotics, and blood pressure medications were all withdrawn in favor of focusing strictly on his comfort. Within days and with his daughter by his side, Elijah Jones died in the hospital listening to his favorite music.

CHAPTER FIVE:
"IF A PICTURE IS WORTH A
THOUSAND WORDS . . ."

As I've said, there are no right and wrong decisions about medical care at the end of life; rather, the value lies in making a fully informed choice. Helen Thompson chose to cut short her medical treatment in favor of time at home with her husband and her books of poetry. In contrast, Elijah Jones was willing to go through just about anything — surgeries, dialysis visits, needles, infections, and catheters — in order to live some more. Statistics interpret many data points, but patients understandably care about only one data point, their own. And Elijah had beaten the statistical lottery.

Whether seriously ill patients are at the point where medical interventions are still helping or at a juncture where interventions only prolong the process of dying is often a personal judgment. The best I could do for Helen and Elijah — and the many other terminally ill patients who came under my care — was make sure they fully understood their treatment options and choices, and that *I* understood where they were on their personal journey in life.

Tours of the ICU and dialysis unit had helped Helen and Elijah, so I began to take all patients and their families on my own personal tour of the hospital, generally at night when the hospital was quieter. If the patients were too unwell to accompany me on tours, even in wheelchairs, then I would take their loved ones through the ICU in their stead.

My tours introduced patients and their families to ventilators, dialysis machines, empty patient rooms with colorful monitors, and, from a distance, the critically ill. I would discuss the general prognoses of patients with various illnesses. What was the likelihood of a patient in the late stages of liver disease surviving CPR? What were the chances that a terminally ill patient with advanced lung disease would have the breathing machine removed? What were some of the other options for a patient with a stroke besides the ICU? These exchanges were some of the most intense and informative I had ever had as a physician. I no longer hid behind the abstract, using unfamiliar medicalese like "life-prolonging interventions" or "comfort as your goal of care." These conversations were tangible and real. The messy clinical details were out in the open. My tours were part show-and-tell and part heart-to-heart. There was not a patient or family member who didn't stop and look at me to say, "Is that what you meant? I had no idea," or, "I heard what you said, but that's not what I imagined," or, "It looks so different on television."

After our tours, some people stuck to their original choices while others changed their minds, but all were more certain about their decisions to pursue all medical interventions, seek a more comfort-oriented approach, or arrange something in between. The ICU journey proved to be transformative, until the ICU nurses put an end to my tour business.

Although the nursing staff felt that there was great educational value in what I was doing and that indeed patients and families were making more informed medical decisions as a result, their priority and loyalty remained first and foremost with their own ICU patients. And they had a legitimate point. Although my tours were always from a distance, one could argue that I was compromising the trust and confidentiality of patients there by bringing other patients or their families on a tour. Almost as quickly as they began, the tours ended.

I had no doubt that these excursions had greatly enhanced my discussions with patients about their own goals for end-of-life care, but how could I circumvent the very real problem of patient confidentiality? If tours were out of the question, what about pictures? I decided to make a video to help my patients and their families understand more clearly what dying in a modern American hospital entails.

Tom Callahan was the youngest of nine children, born into a strict Irish Catholic working-class family in the Dorchester section of Boston. He and Ted Kennedy were born within months of each other in the same ward at St. Margaret's Hospital in Dorchester, little more than a hop, skip, and a jump from the hustle and bustle of downtown Boston. But over the next seventy years, the two men could not have followed more different paths.

Whereas Kennedy attended the prestigious Milton Academy and Harvard College, Tom completed a high school equivalency degree at a local community college. Kennedy, from one of America's most esteemed families, went on to a high-profile life in politics, and by the end of his nearly fifty years in the nation's upper house he was known as "the Lion of the Senate." Tom worked as a plumber, toiling in his blue-collar neighborhood.

But now that both had surpassed Psalm 90:10's promise of threescore years and ten, their paths converged once again. Tom and Ted were both suffering from advanced brain cancer, and both faced many of the same decisions about the course of their medical care.

Tom, who never lost the disciplined habits of his upbringing, always arrived punctually for his appointment with his oncologist, and he began each session with a communal prayer for himself, his family, and his doctor. "So teach us to number our days, that we may apply our hearts unto wisdom." He was consistently flanked by his guardian angels: his wife of forty-eight years, Teresa, on one side and his older sister Agnes on the other.

The pair faithfully attended all his medical appointments and buoyed his spirits with their fierce optimism. Nevertheless, Tom tempered the family's hopeful outlook about his prognosis with a thoughtful realism and pragmatism all his own — qualities that made him the ideal audience for the premiere of my first medical video, more than two years in the making.

Eight months before I met Tom, he'd been diagnosed with glioblastoma multiforme, the same tumor that cost Helen her memory and her life. The onslaught of radiation and medicines had temporarily staved off the aggressive growth of Tom's brain tumor but he was weaker by the day, increasingly less able to sing his favorite Irish songs at the pub with his buddies, accompanied by a fiddle and uilleann pipes. Over the past twenty-four hours, Tom's headaches had worsened; he was vomiting, and he was becoming dehydrated. He had come to the hospital for intravenous fluids, which would help with his dehydration and headaches but would not have an effect on his overall prognosis. Tom needed to decide how he wished to live out his remaining days.

He looked comfortable. He was resting in the hospital bed with his wife on one side, holding his hand and softly singing to comfort him, while his sister was on the other side praying with rosary beads.

"I'm sorry to interrupt," I said, feeling a bit ill at ease for intruding on an intimate moment that transcended the brutal realities of Tom's illness.

I introduced myself, and Teresa and Agnes

immediately rose to shake my hand. "Hello, Doctor. I am Tom's wife, Teresa, and this is Agnes, Tom's sister. And this is Tom."

"Hey, Doc." Tom was tired but comfortable.

"How you feeling, buddy?" I asked. The first question I asked a new patient was always the hardest for me, since it set the tone for the rest of the interview. "How you feeling, buddy?" seemed just right for Tom.

To calm my own anxieties, I focused on the usual litany of medical questions. Where was the pain? When did it begin? What was the pain like? Any associated symptoms? Any patterns or things that change the pain? On a scale of one to ten, with ten being the worst, how bad is it? By the time I finished my history and physical exam, I was calm enough to start asking the really tough questions.

"Tom, I want to have a conversation with you about how you want to live and what gives you happiness in life."

"Am I gonna die, Doc?"

"We're all going to die someday, Tom. Have you ever spoken with your doctor about your prognosis?"

"He never raised the issue of dying with me." Tom was little different from most seriously ill patients.

"Tom, I don't want to talk to you about dying. I want to talk to you about living. I want to know how you want to live. What gives you happiness and joy?"

"I love being home with my wife, our kids, and grandkids, and my sister. And I love singing my Irish songs. I wouldn't want to go on if I couldn't sing with my buddies."

"Tom, tell me what you understand about how things are going with your brain tumor."

"Not so well. I think it's still doing its thing. I'm growing a watermelon in my head, Doc." He smiled, but he barely had the strength for a modest chuckle.

I knew the grim statistics, the cold hard facts of glioblastoma multiforme. Tom's days were clearly numbered. Not single-digit numbered, but he would be lucky if he lived more than three more months. "We need to have a discussion about where we go from here," I told him. "I want to focus on how you can live with this illness on your own terms."

"I want to know what my choices are, Doc."

"Okay, let's review them. But to get the conversation going, I want to first watch an educational video with you. It will review some of the choices that we can talk about.

Is that okay?"

"Whatever you say."

With the trepidation no doubt shared by all first-time producers, I pushed "play" on the video for Tom, Teresa, and Agnes.

Creating the video Tom was about to see was not easy. Fortunately, my early dabbling in filmmaking provided a good starting point. My godfather was an amateur film-maker in New York City. From a very young age, I was exposed to the process of filming and editing in his makeshift studio in his living room, where I would be in charge of splicing film ends together and gathering the discarded pieces of negative film from the cutting-room floor. When I was a teen-ager, my parents bought me a secondhand sixteen-millimeter movie camera to nurture my interest.

My interest in film continued throughout high school and college, but it wasn't until medical school in the 1990s that my pursuit of documentary filmmaking took off in earnest. Despite the workload of my medi-cal studies I took a seminar that focused on what was at the time a revolutionary new way of filmmaking, one that did not rely on the cumbersome process of splicing nega-tive films and sorting through discarded strips of film on the cutting-room floor: Digital Filmmaking and the Documentary Film Tradition. Little did I know then how truly life-altering that seminar would be for me and, quite a few years later, for Tom and all of my other patients.

That seminar reminded me of the single most important lesson I'd learned from my godfather: A good deal of thinking and interviewing needed to be accomplished before framing the first shot. I applied that same approach to the production of my new medical video.

For an entire year prior to filming, I interviewed scores of seriously ill patients and their families, as well as loved ones of deceased patients, to understand what the experience of making decisions about medical care was like. Their insights were astounding.

"No one explained to me what all that medical jargon really meant," one elderly patient with advanced heart disease told me. "You doctors don't speak English." A middle-aged patient with aggressive cancer told me, "I wanted to discuss my options with my physician, but she was more interested in talking about what combination of surgery, chemo, and radiation worked best. She didn't bother to ask if I were interested in any of the above." And perhaps most telling was the refrain that I heard from numerous family members: "I don't think anyone ever had a conversation with us or asked what we wanted."

At the same time, I began talking with clinicians including oncologists, ICU doctors, cardiologists, ethicists, geriatricians, surgeons, palliative care doctors, medical residents, nurses, social workers, and chaplains. As I'd seen before, some doctors never had a conversation with their patients about end-of-life care. For those who did, each had his or her own way of broaching the issue and discussing care at the end of life, especially when it came to CPR: the actual mechanics of it, the prognosis, the complications, and even whether or not CPR was appropriate for some patients with a serious illness. But it was not simply a matter of differences in style. Some clinicians entirely misstated or overlooked some basic and essential facts, and there was considerable variation in which aspects of CPR were presented to patients.

A few physicians focused on the likelihood of a patient with advanced disease surviving CPR and walking out of the hospital, while others never mentioned the odds of surviving the procedure. Some framed the discussion vividly: "We would punch you on your chest and crack your ribs." Others described the process using toned-down language, "We would push on your chest vigorously." Perhaps most concerning was the abundance of doctors who depended on medicalese, jargon that only a person with clinical training and experience would understand. Clinicians routinely pepper their patients with technical terms: cardioversion, arrhythmia, ventricular fibrillation, pulseless electrical activity, intubation, ventilators, central line, epinephrine, cardiac arrest, asystole, and hypoxia.

It was remarkable that all these clinicians worked in the same health care system, and yet all had very different discussions with patients — which may have led to very different medical care. A patient's decision-making will be influenced by which doctor admits him or her to the hospital or is assigned to a patient during admission, and by that doctor's ability or inability to have an informed discussion about treatment options.

Despite all the variability, however, there was a common theme that emerged from my interviews with patients and clinicians. Almost everyone conceptualized the choices for medical care at the end of life along a spectrum with three general options. At one end was a full code, a full-court press, where the main goal of medical care was to prolong life with any medical intervention available regardless of whether the success rate was slim or the intervention caused great suffering. Taras, Nonna, and Elijah experienced all the risks and benefits of the entire arsenal of medical interventions. At the other end of the spectrum was a comfort-oriented approach. The focus was on making sure a patient was not in pain and the priority was to remain outside of the hospital, ideally at home, with appropriate hospice care. Helen's medical care had focused on her comfort.

Everything else was somewhere in between. This middle-of-the-road approach didn't include overly invasive treatments (no CPR and breathing machines), nor was it entirely focused on comfort-oriented measures. The goal was maintaining basic functions like walking, talking, eating, seeing, hearing, and thinking.

Based on patients' and physicians' suggestions, these three choices became: Life-Prolonging Care, Limited Medical Care, and Comfort Care. Now I needed to find images to illustrate these three options to patients and their families.

During the next year or so, a group of clinicians from my research group and I got permission from patients to film them in order to educate others. To our surprise, patients, families, and medical staff not only gave consent for us to film them but also wondered why such a video was not already available. One of the most poignant moments came when the daughter of an elderly patient who was connected to a breathing machine said, "I wouldn't be in this situation if someone had had a conversation with me about Mom's options and if I had understood what I was agreeing to." Many family members shared with us similar stories and sentiments.

Once we had the go-ahead, we filmed everywhere: at patients' homes, in the ICU, at skilled nursing facilities, in the dialysis unit, even in the operating room. Our goal was to capture the essence of Helen Thompson's and Elijah Jones's tours on film. CPR, ventilators, the ICU, dialysis, hospital wards, and hospice — nothing was left to the imagination. These real-life images would serve as a corrective to the misleading ones perpetrated by Hollywood.

We wanted to create a video that would empower patients and be beyond reproach from medical colleagues, ethicists, and, of course, patients. That meant there could be no bias, no matter how unintentional, that might subtly push patients to choose one of the three available options over the others. Any hint of trying to nudge patients toward any one direction would discredit the whole project.

Selecting which shots to include in the video was a painstaking and excruciatingly slow process that addressed the concerns and critiques of our expert reviewers, both doctors and patients. Doctors are by nature defensive when it comes to talking about death, which is of little surprise in a profession where death's presence is the elephant in the room. What we didn't expect was that they could be more finicky than professional film critics. Patients were no different. They, too, were more than willing to give our team sharp reviews of the video that would make most wince. It took us two years to produce one short video. But we needed our critics' unanimous agreement that our creation was both fair and impartial.

Two significant changes were made to the video based on reviewers' comments. First we deleted all patient testimonials. In an effort to remain impartial, we had filmed various patients and family members explaining why they had made a particular decision.

For instance, we had one family member of a patient explain why her deceased father had decided to remain a full code to the very end; another patient, a nurse with widely metastatic cancer, offered her thoughts on why comfort care was the best choice for her. Each of these gripping vignettes was memorable and powerful, which is why in their wisdom patients and doctors wanted them excluded: The testimonials were too prejudicial to the decision-making process. Here, complete objectivity was the gold standard.

The second recommendation was to edit out scenes that were not considered strictly medical. We had filmed an ICU nurse combing and then trimming the hair of a patient who was intubated and on a breathing machine. In another scene, a medical aide helped a patient shave. Our critics, however, effectively argued that these scenes misconstrued the primary goals of the three categories and were distracting. They, too, were cut.

After much editing, reworking, and rewriting of the script, our critics agreed that the final video was impartial and a fair portrayal. After we left the editing room and returned to the hospital, the team had to decide on the first patient to see the video.

The decision was left to me. I chose Tom.

"If a picture is worth a thousand words, a video is worth hundreds of thousands," Tom said when the video ended. "Now that I've seen my options, I'll take comfort care, Doc." Tom's wife, Teresa, and his sister Agnes began to absorb the import of his decision.

"Are you sure, Tommy? I'll support you in whatever you choose," Teresa told him.

"If the cancer ain't getting better and my chances are slim, why would I want to be put on all those machines? No thanks. I value my time with my family, not hospitals. We've had a great run, Doc. Let me be at home with my family."

"Whatever you say, Tommy," Teresa said, tears slipping down her cheeks.

"It's okay with me, little brother. I don't think anyone wants you to be on the machines in the video if things get really bad," added Agnes.

I looked at Tom and said, "It'll be all right. We'll go down this road together."

As I got up to leave, Agnes and Teresa took hold of each of Tom's hands. I left the room wondering what I would have wanted if I were in Tom's shoes.

One month later, Tom died at home surrounded by Teresa, Agnes, the rest of his family, and his Boston buddies. Ted Kennedy died not long after Tom. It was reported that on the day Kennedy died, he was eating ice cream and watching his favorite James Bond movie at home with his family. Although they lived starkly different lives after leaving the delivery ward at St. Margaret's, both men found themselves in similar circumstances when the end came, their lives converging once again, at least symbolically, where they had begun.

The video helped Tom understand his options, have The Conversation with me, and decide what he desired at the final stage of his life. But I had to be sure that the video would help other patients as well. Before any innovation is introduced routinely into patient care, an objective experiment must be performed to determine whether the new treatment is helpful to patients compared to the standard of care, that is, the current treatment. A randomized trial of the video would be the only currency that doctors would accept or trust.

In order to determine whether or not the video helped patients with a serious illness make decisions that they were comfortable with, some oncologists and I decided to recruit fifty patients with advanced brain cancer into a randomized controlled trial. Once the oncologists agreed that a patient was eligible for the study, he or she would be randomly assigned by computer to either the intervention or the control group, ensuring that the results would remain impartial.

The patients in the control group made decisions about their end-of-life care after a verbal discussion only, without the use of the video. The verbal discussion used a script that we had created of what an idealized conversation with a doctor would be like. Patients who had only a verbal discussion made the following choices using the three categories of care: About a quarter chose Life-Prolonging Care, that is, an all-out effort with all available interventions; another quarter decided on Comfort Care, preferring to focus on their symptoms with hospice care at home; and around half opted for Limited Medical Care — essentially somewhere in the middle. These results were very much in line with my own experience treating patients with advanced cancer.

The patients in the intervention group made decisions about their medical care after receiving the same idealized conversation script and after they viewed the video. This group's choices were quite different and told a powerful story. After viewing the video, none of the patients chose Life-Prolonging Care, just a handful opted for Limited Medical Care, and the overwhelming majority (92 percent) decided on Comfort Care.

But the differences between the two groups were not only in patients' expressed choices; patients who viewed the video also had more knowledge about their choices. As part of the study, we asked the control group patients a series of true-false questions before and after we spoke to them to gauge their understanding of each of the three choices available to them. We asked the intervention group patients the same series of questions before and after we spoke to them and showed them the video. Some of the questions included:

Once you tell your doctor what kind of medical care you want if your cancer becomes very advanced, you cannot change your wishes in the future.
(False)

Comfort Care is a type of medical care that can only be provided for patients with

advanced cancer living in hospice.
(False)

CPR is a medical procedure that is done on patients whose heart stops beating in an attempt to restart their heart.
(True)

Most patients with advanced cancer who survive CPR and being placed on a breathing machine have few complications from these procedures.
(False)

How many patients with advanced cancer that get CPR in the hospital survive and get to leave the hospital: A. almost all (more than 90 percent); B. about half (about 50 percent); or C. few (fewer than 10 percent).
(C)

Patients who saw the video answered more questions correctly than those who did not. More than 80 percent of patients stated they were "very comfortable" using the video, and the remaining said they were "somewhat comfortable." But perhaps most important, all of the patients who watched the video said they would recommend it to others. It is one thing to introduce medical concepts in the abstract, and completely another thing to show documentary evidence of just what these concepts mean in real life.

These results were published in 2010 in the *Journal of Clinical Oncology,* and as significant as they were, they also raised new questions, chiefly whether the video could be applied with similar results to patients with other advanced cancers. We were determined to find out.

Our research team's next study recruited one hundred fifty patients with all different types of advanced cancer: lung, colon, breast, and liver cancers, among others. All were critically ill and unlikely to survive more than a few months, a year at best. Since many of these patients were in critical condition, we used a shortened version of the original video to focus only on CPR. This study narrowed the decision patients would make to a single one: Would you or would you not want physicians to attempt CPR if your heart stops beating?

Once again, we randomized half of the patients with advanced cancer to the video group and half to the control group. In the control group, nearly half of patients with a serious illness wished to have CPR attempted. Among those who viewed the video, just 20 percent preferred to undergo CPR. Our study was presented at the largest meeting of oncologists in the world, the American Society of Clinical Oncology, and published in 2013 in the *Journal of Clinical Oncology.*

My research group has replicated these findings in numerous clinical trials over the past few years, including in patients with different illnesses (e.g., dementia) and in different clinical settings (e.g., outpatient, inpatient, nursing home, ICU). The research suggests that patients make better-informed decisions using a video because they see possible procedures and interventions with their own eyes.

An interesting finding from our studies is that a video also inspires more patients to have The Conversation with their doctors. Today, the typical doctor-patient encounter follows the dominant mode of education in which the teacher (doctor) has most of the power and knowledge in the relationship. The doctor seeks to transfer knowledge to the patient (student), which unfortunately induces passivity and disempowerment on the part of the patient. Instead, imagine encounters in which patients are prepared to engage in shared decision-making by videos that provide simple information that offer them their options for medical care. Activating the patient with the information to have a dialogue with the physician promotes patient-centeredness and engagement. It also "flips" the dynamic in the doctor-patient relationship, in which the patient starts to wield some of the power (knowledge).

The effectiveness of videos is not unique to medicine. Consider how videos are revolutionizing the way children are learning throughout the world due in large part to one man, Salman "Sal" Khan. In the summer of 2004, Sal started remotely tutoring his seventh-grade cousin, who was having trouble in math, using Google's sketchpad and the telephone. By 2006, he was recording lectures on YouTube. These videos became so wildly popular that thousands of students began viewing them. In 2008, Sal left his position at a hedge fund and created Khan Academy, a nonprofit foundation.

Today, Khan Academy is radically changing the way students learn. Children all over the world can obtain a top-notch education using the more than 2,200 videos that have been created on subjects in math, science, or the humanities. About one million students use the videos monthly, and school districts in California have already incorporated the videos into their curricula. The videos represent a paradigm shift, a radical rethinking of pedagogy and education more generally.

Khan Academy's videos not only have the potential to turn the student-teacher relationship on its head, but might actually break its neck. It is becoming increasingly unacceptable to have substandard teachers offer students recycled lectures when the best teachers are available online giving riveting lectures. Students are embracing digital technology — and why should they expect anything less from the education system in the digital age?

Patients and families should likewise change their expectations of doctors and hospitals in the digital age. Indeed, videos have the potential to reinvent medicine and to reengineer the patient-doctor relationship. With videos, patients can obtain the information they need to make informed decisions with tools that empower them and allow them to deliberate about decisions at a pace that they dictate. They can visualize and imagine health care options more accurately with video aids that provide readily understandable information. Then the health care system's most scarce resource

— time spent with physicians — can be dedicated to asking questions after patients have had time to digest and absorb the needed information.

Using videos to supplement patient-doctor discussions can also help standardize exchanges between doctors and patients across the country, cutting out varieties in style, personality, candor, and approach in individual physicians. As you'll recall from earlier in the chapter, doctors sometimes omit or misstate facts in conversations about medical interventions. Videos help standardize the information shared.

It is important to note that the role of the video is to augment — not supplant — the patient-doctor relationship. Doctor communication remains the bedrock of the patient-doctor relationship; videos only provide general information about levels of care and treatment options. Videos help patients prepare to talk to their providers and understand their choices in broad terms. For applicability to specific patients, doctors provide the requisite knowledge of a patient's medical condition, likely prognosis, and outcomes. Video decision aids explain risks and benefits and assist patients in identifying their individual values and preferences. They present information in a structured way and provide the evidence patients need to assess their options.

Video education in medicine has been successfully used and in wide circulation for more than twenty years in many clinical contexts beyond end-of-life care. Hospitals and clinics have been implementing medical videos for surgical operations and complex medical decisions into routine medical care. In 2009, Group Health Cooperative, a network of physicians and clinics for more than half a million patients in Washington State, started a massive effort to change the culture of care by incorporating twelve video decision aids for medical decisions into clinical practice in six areas: orthopedics, cardiology, urology, women's health, breast cancer, and back care. Thousands of Group Health patients making decisions about medical care regarding herniated disks, breast cancer, uterine fibroids, prostate cancer, osteoarthritis of the hip and knee, heart disease, and many other conditions use videos to better inform themselves of their options. And Group Heath's efforts are paying off.

In 2013, a team of their researchers published a study in the journal *Health Affairs* of one of the largest implementations of video decision aids to date. It detailed the enhancement in decision quality for patients by using video. Video decision aids allow patients to be more actively involved in decision-making, more knowledgeable about the facts, and less uncertain regarding their preferences. This leads to medical care that is consistent with patient values.

In today's rushed doctor visit, a physician may often not have the time to adequately cover all the information needed for the patient to make an informed decision at the end of life. Video support tools help ensure that patients and families get the details they need to make decisions consistent with their beliefs and goals. And there is ample precedent for such interventions that remind busy physicians of needed medical care.

Physicians use checklists to remind themselves of the information and best practices at their fingertips. For instance, many intensive care units have checklists to remind physicians of proper sterile techniques for inserting central lines; and most surgical operating rooms use checklists to reinforce accepted safety practices and to foster better communication and teamwork. Videos are essentially visual checklists that help provide patients and families with the necessary information about their medical options at the end of life. If a physician is hurried or forgets to provide some of the information a patient needs to make an informed decision, a video supplies the essential information — and it can be reviewed as many times as a patient wishes, without a need to hurry. A video may also empower a patient to press a physician to have The Conversation, if needed.

One concern sometimes raised regarding the use of videos is that they could possibly usurp the patient-doctor relationship, instead of opening up a discussion regarding end-of-life preferences. Some argue that physicians may be more inclined to have patients view a video rather than have a lengthy conversation with them about end-of-life choices. Thus, instead of reinforcing The Conversation, videos may replace The Conversation, and even enable the doctor to avoid the topic altogether. Although this argument may appear to have some merit, in practice it has not been a significant problem, as videos have been successfully used in many medical settings.

Nonetheless, an objective study suggesting that a proposed change is better than the existing standard of care is only the beginning. The introduction and widespread acceptance of that change — in this case, the use of videos that illustrate the three standards of end-of-life care — is no simple matter. Clinical medicine is inherently a conservative science. Changes occur at a snail's pace, and for good reason: Lives are on the line. Sometimes what works well in the lab may not pan out in practice. The history of medicine is, unfortunately, marred by recommendations that were hastily enacted without the requisite level of proof.

Medicine aspires to universality, but some of today's medical truths will be disproved within a few generations, just as others are discarded by the time a student completes his lengthy medical education. As medical advances are made, some of the previous threads of knowledge must be unraveled. Among physicians, the price of knowledge is the recognition of previous errors in judgment. For my part, a very real test of the effectiveness and impact of the video occurred unexpectedly close to home.

CHAPTER SIX:
COMING HOME

The medical team met in the cafeteria to review the new patients who were admitted from the previous night, as we did at seven each morning. My beeper suddenly went off, but I wasn't being paged by the hospital. The callback number was my mother's in New York City. With much trepidation, I immediately returned the page.

"Mom? Is everything okay?"

"Your father had a stroke. Come home." My mother's tremulous voice was drowned out by the din of activity and I could barely hear her.

The rest of that morning is a blur. My residents and I reviewed our new patients and then I arranged for a senior colleague to cover me for the next two days. I called my wife, who was at work, and told her that I was heading to New York immediately. I then called our young daughter just to hear her voice. At these moments, there is nothing more reassuring than hearing your child on the telephone. I'm sure my mother felt the same way when we talked earlier that morning.

I tried to stay calm, but my heart was racing. As a senior physician, I had admitted scores of stroke patients, and a kaleidoscope of faces bombarded my memory. This time, the patient was my father, but I had the same essential questions.

What type of stroke did he have, hemorrhagic or thromboembolic? What did the CT or MRI show? What were his initial symptoms, and when did they begin? Did he have an abrupt onset of impaired cerebral function with generalized symptoms, or did he present with specific neurologic deficits? Are the doctors sure it was a stroke? Seizures, syncope, migraine, and hypoglycemia can often mimic acute ischemia. Had they considered a broad enough range of potential diagnoses?

Dad was already on a host of medications for his heart failure, high cholesterol, and diabetes. Perhaps he had missed a dose of one of them and this mimicked a stroke? Did the doctors have access to his medications and his medical history? I reviewed the questions again and again as I sped to New York City, trying to beat the afternoon rush-hour traffic and hoping not to get pulled over.

I almost missed the exit for the Triborough Bridge heading into the city. It had been recently renamed RFK Bridge in honor of Robert F. Kennedy. Even though I had taken this route many times, TRIBOROUGH BRIDGE EXIT — PAY TOLL was my visual reminder to get off at the exit, and that cue was no longer there. Instead, RFK BRIDGE was now printed in large white letters on the burnished green road sign.

When I was a young kid growing up in the city, my dad and I would play "Name That Bridge." He would give me the boroughs, and I would have to name the bridge that connected them. My father would always give me hints if I needed them, rattling off landmarks as if he had grown up in New York City and not in the tiny village in Greece that I visited during summers.

"Brooklyn and Manhattan."

"Brooklyn Bridge!"

"And . . . if Brooklyn has a bridge, shouldn't the other borough have one named after it, too?"

"Manhattan Bridge!"

"And which bridge connects Queens, the Bronx, and Manhattan?"

"Triborough Bridge!" The vibrations of

his stentorian voice still resonated in my ears after all these years. It would take some time for me to get used to the bridge's new name.

I left it behind me and made for the hospital, a large academic medical center not very different from my own. It was a motley assortment of buildings constructed over decades or even centuries, with ultramodern glass wings attached to turn-of-the-century neoclassical buildings, a mash-up of architectural styles. But there was a beauty in traveling through the labyrinthine hallways of the disjointed buildings. I hurried to the Neuro-ICU in the newest wing of the hospital, and in some ways, I was traveling through a medical time machine traversing the progress of modern technology.

If it had been just a decade or two earlier, my father would have been dead before he'd even had this stroke. Thanks to medical advances, he had survived two heart attacks and was being aggressively treated for diabetes. Yesterday's miracles soon become today's standard of care; and technological discoveries I had only read about in medical school were now standard at hospitals across the country.

As soon as I arrived in the unit, my

father's nurse filled me in on what had happened. My father had some weakness on one side of his body, and a CT scan had suggested a stroke. He had immediately been brought to the Neuro-ICU for closer observation, and luckily, his left side was slowly improving. I asked the nurse to page the medical resident while I made my way to my dad's room.

Mom was sitting at my sleeping father's bedside, holding his hand. He was wearing a nasal cannula, which supplied him with oxygen, and he had an intravenous line in each arm. I was surprised by just how normal he appeared. The monitor that beeped with each heartbeat showed that his blood pressure was mildly elevated but stable, his heart rate excellent, and his oxygen saturation normal. I breathed a sigh of relief. Dad was out of imminent danger. I now could attend to my mother.

"I was scared," she told me, weeping gently. "It was so fast. I forgot all of my things at home."

"It's okay, Mom. Everything will be okay. Dad's gonna do fine. His vital signs are fine. He'll pull through." As I heard myself say "vital signs," I immediately regretted it. What are vital signs to my mother, or to any patient's spouse? My role here was not to play doctor, but instead to be a supportive family member, a son. I hugged my mom as a doctor entered the room.

"I am sorry to interrupt, Dr. Volandes. It's Dr. Mark Davidson, the medical resident. We met last year when your dad came in with heart failure."

I shook Mark's hand. Had it already been a year? I had lost track of the number of times my dad had been admitted to the hospital. It had begun five years earlier with his first heart attack, followed by a subsequent one, and then multiple admissions for heart failure and diabetes. With each admission, I would get to know the new batch of residents. Acquainting myself with residents was my own strategy for organizing the disruption and chaos that disease wrought on my family.

"Your dad is stable. His limb weakness is improving. His vital signs are good and we'll keep checking for hyperglycemia. He's scheduled to have a repeat head CT at twenty-four hours. Neuro checks every thirty minutes."

"Thanks, Mark. And thanks for everything you're doing for my dad."

"The team reviewed the case with our senior doctor and we just finished rounding. I have the films up on the computer

181

screen if you would like to review them with me."

"Maybe later." Although I insisted on reviewing the films of my patients firsthand, I was more interested in staying close to my mom and dad.

"Mrs. Volandes, can I get you anything?" the resident asked.

"No, thank you, Mark."

"There is one thing that I'd like to confirm with the two of you if that's all right. After Mr. Volandes came to the unit and was stabilized, he was still confused. I had a conversation with Mrs. Volandes about his goals of care and code status. I just want to confirm that Mr. Volandes is now DNR — Do Not Resuscitate. He does not wish to have CPR if his heart should stop beating, nor does he want to be placed on a ventilator if he is unable to breathe on his own, correct? I just want to make sure because when he was admitted to my service last year he was a full code."

"That's right. Those are my husband's wishes."

DNR? Do not resuscitate? Do not resuscitate Dad? How could that be? It was as if I was hearing DNR for the very first time, even though I had written DNR orders for hundreds of my patients and did not think twice about it. But this was different; this was my father.

"Dr. Volandes?" Mark asked.

I was frozen. I turned my gaze toward my mother, and then to Mark.

"Yes, whatever my mom and father agreed upon."

"Good. Just wanted to confirm. The repeat head CT won't be done until the morning. Perhaps you both should head home and rest. I will call you if anything changes. Great to see you again, Dr. Volandes. Please let me know if I can be of any additional help."

I called my sister and brother to update them on our father's condition. Even though they lived closer to my parents than I did, my mother always called me first during a medical emergency; I was the doctor in the family. I assured them that Dad was stable, and told them to come to the hospital the following day.

As Mom and I drove home over the Brooklyn Bridge, I could almost hear Dad's heavily accented voice rattle off more landmarks and hints. "Brooklyn and Staten Island . . . Verrazano!"

By the time we arrived home, it was well past midnight. Things were in disarray. My mom and I began cleaning and sorting

183

things in the house; neither of us could sleep. I could only think of three letters: *D-N-R.*

"Mom, did you and Dad discuss things recently, about his DNR? I must admit, it came as a complete shock to me."

"Right after Thanksgiving."

"Thanksgiving?"

"We were going to discuss it with you, but we hadn't yet had the chance. Look, at some point you say enough is enough. He's not giving up or anything, but going to the hospital for medicines and checkups is one thing. Having people pound on his chest and put him on a breathing machine is another. And maybe he wouldn't even come back home after all that? It would be a nightmare." She stopped and sighed.

Was it the emotional exhaustion? Or simply the acknowledgment of our own mortality?

"But if he has a good quality of life . . ."

"We're older now and we've had a good life — better than most. But if we reach a point where we can't enjoy the things that give us happiness, then don't draw things out by putting us on those machines. You'll understand when you get to this point. Once we reviewed again the video you e-mailed, we made up our minds."

Her explanation was reasonable. She understood CPR and the slim likelihood of my father surviving the procedure given his advanced illnesses, and she understood the many risks and small benefits of other life-prolonging interventions. This was exactly the level of understanding I hoped all my patients and their families would achieve. My parents were the perfect patients: They had paid attention to each detail and were informed about their choices. So why was it so hard for me to accept DNR for Dad?

"We reviewed the video together a bunch of times," she continued. "Stopping, replaying, discussing . . . We thought the best decision would be nothing too much, nothing aggressive. It's the right decision. It's the right decision for our family. Now help me clean. Easter is coming up and I want to make sure the house is ready before everyone comes over for dinner."

I kept cleaning the house for the next couple of hours until I was exhausted. Perhaps it was the late hour or maybe it was my physical weariness, but my thinking was muddled. "It's the right decision for our family" kept reverberating in my mind.

By three A.M., I was brushing my teeth and heading toward my childhood bedroom. The Eagle Scout badges and science fair trophies were angled on the dresser, exactly as I'd left them when I went off to college. Mom insisted on preserving the room, even keeping the boxy Apple Macintosh computer and my first sixteen-millimeter movie camera. During the holidays, my daughter slept on the tiny twin bed with the overwashed Batman and Robin bedsheets that I had slept on throughout childhood. I could not imagine a more comfortable place to rest my exhausted frame, and it was the perfect therapy for my own anxiety.

Doctors fear the death of a parent, all the more so when we admit a patient who reminds us of our own father or mother. The outlines of Taras's immigrant story differed little from my father's: They both came from faraway lands, worked hard in blue-collar jobs, and lived the American Dream. Stories about Nonna's pasta e fagioli prompted memories of my mother perfecting her Greek recipes. How many elderly males with a heart attack (or diabetes, or a stroke) had I admitted over the years that reminded me of my father? How many elderly women's hearts had I listened to that had led me to a fleeting thought of what my mother's heart sounded like and how long it would keep beating? When I looked into the eyes of Taras, Nonna, Miguel, Helen, Elijah, Tom, or any of my patients with an ophthalmoscope, I was also staring right into the deeper recesses of my own soul and facing the mortality of my parents — and, in some ways, my own.

That night my anxiety manifested in a dream. It was one I'd had before. I was in my first year on the wards as a medical resident. The gray had not yet arrived in my hair, and I was back to being an eager young doctor. "Code Blue!" blared and I raced through the hospital, running faster and stronger than I could remember ever running. There was no need to compose myself as I had while a young doctor; I had run a code many times since residency. I knew the medicines and the procedures instinctually. My body in the dream may have been that of my younger self, but my mind had more than a decade of experience treating patients. I stood at the foot of the patient's bed and took charge, secure in my knowledge and experience as a seasoned physician. Adrenaline was coursing through my veins, but my pulse remained steady.

A nurse was performing chest compressions, someone else was pumping air into the patient's lungs with a green breathing bag, and another was administering lifesaving drugs while simultaneously monitoring the code. I was in control.

"Please stop compressions, and let's check for a pulse."

And then somehow I lost my composure and my heart began to race. As the nurse removed the green breathing bag, I could finally make out the face of the patient. It was my father. I cried out.

I awoke, drenched in sweat, as my beeper went off. My heart was pounding. I threw off the bedsheets. Where was I? Was I still in a dream?

My beeper went off again. It was seven A.M., and I didn't recognize the number. Who would be paging me from a New York phone number?

"Dr. Volandes, it's Mark. Sorry to bother you."

"What's wrong? Is anything wrong with my dad?"

"He's fine. The repeat head CT shows no further changes. He's doing better. He's not able to move his lower extremities fully, but I'll have physical therapy swing by. Just wanted to call and let you know."

"Okay. Sorry, I thought . . . We're heading over in the next couple of hours. I'll let my mother know. Thanks." How many times had I called family members in the early hours of the morning to tell them news of their loved one? Now I was on the other end of the receiver. Luckily, the news this time was good.

It was a frigid March morning and my mother and I quickly bundled ourselves in overcoats and joined the slow-moving traffic over the Brooklyn Bridge. We entered the hospital and made our way to the transparent glass-walled wing of the Neuro-ICU. Dad was seated in his bed drinking some soup from a straw.

"This food stinks!" he complained. "No salt. Who makes soup without salt?"

We both hugged him. If he was complaining about food, then he was back to his normal self. Except for the unsteadiness in his gait, his mind and body were left untouched by the stroke. And with physical rehabilitation, he was expected to make a complete recovery. Physicians would consider him one more example of the technological miracle of modern medicine, but to our family he was just back to being Dad.

My siblings arrived and the disruption and chaos slowly loosened its hold on us. By that afternoon, Mark and the medical team had transferred my father out of the Neuro-ICU. He was to undergo a few days of physical therapy in the hospital and then would be moved to a rehabilitation facility for a few weeks. If all went well, Dad would be home by Easter. I felt confident enough about my father's prognosis that I said good-bye and headed back to Boston.

As I drove, the inexorable march of the future hit me: One day, likely soon, there would be a holiday dinner first without my father, and then eventually without my mother. I rolled down my car window to pay the toll for the renamed RFK Bridge, crying openly as the frigid March wind buffeted my face.

It was frigid again as I arrived at work at five the next morning, determined to put the difficult times of my emergency trip to New York behind me and catch up on the latest admissions to the hospital. I didn't know it then, but I was about to meet the patient whose death before my eyes would confirm my growing unease about medical care in today's America and launch this memoir in a bid to help change it.

Hospitals in the early morning can be eerie places. The hallways are blinding with their bright fluorescent lights and white-washed walls. Few personnel roam the halls except for the occasional transport staffer who is wheeling a patient on a gurney to a room from the emergency department.

Apart from the hum of a ventilation shaft or the ring of an elevator, the hospital is silent, which can be alarming, so unlike the usual cacophony of hospital disturbances. It had been many years since I had last roamed the hospital hallways in the wee hours of the morning, not since residency.

Melissa, a nurse working on the medicine floor, did a double take when she saw me at the nurses' station. "Dr. Volandes, what are you doing on Greenberg Five at this ungodly hour?" One would not be surprised to see a resident at this time of day, but a senior doctor was out of place.

"Any chance you want to review some of the new patients from the last two days?" Checking in with the night nurse was an important lesson I'd learned in residency. The overnight briefing, or "sign-out," was officially the responsibility of the night physician, but an early rundown was always helpful.

Melissa reviewed her list of patients. "Let's see. I have G.W., A.D., T.C., J.V., A.T. Most of them were pretty quiet except for L.B., Lillian Badakian. She's our thirty-two-year-old patient with widely metastatic breast cancer, status post–bilateral mastectomy, radiotherapy, and failed first- and second-line chemotherapies. But her more urgent issue is that she's in excruciating pain with metastases to her bone, despite being on large doses of pain meds. Her blood pressure is tenuous and her heart rate has been all over the place. And, she's a full code."

"Seriously? A full code?"

"Full code," Melissa repeated.

"Can the patient make decisions on her own?"

"If you catch her at the right time. The poor thing is always in agony. The team gave her morphine to help with the pain, and we started her on a patient-controlled analgesia IV so that she could self-medicate as well, but she's not using it. She insists on not being overmedicated so that she can remain alert and speak with her husband. He is always by her side. Her three kids, all boys, are at home with the grandparents. It breaks my heart to see her in so much pain. This is so sad."

Why, I wondered, would she subject her cancer-ravaged body to the brutality of CPR and other emergency procedures and be tethered to a hospital bed when medical science could offer her virtually no hope of survival beyond a few weeks, or even days? Wouldn't she rather spend these last, precious moments as comfortable as possible with her husband and three young sons? Determined to find out, I read through Lillian's medical records. Three generations of Badakian mothers had already succumbed to this horrible disease. Her family was hoping for a new ending this time, but I knew that her tale was likely following the same tragic story line.

I approached Lillian's room and gently opened the door to see if she was awake. Before I could peer inside the room, the haunting sound of a clarinet accompanied by chants escaped from the doorway. I instantly recognized the Byzantine-like chant from my childhood days of attending church; the monophonic vocals differed little from the ones my parents would play during Easter. The music was simultaneously plaintive and soul-stirring. Through the music, I could hear Lillian's soft whimpers. Her husband was kneeling by her bedside, whispering to her and clasping her hands.

"I'm sorry to interrupt. My name is Angelo Volandes. I'm one of the doctors in charge." Calling myself Dr. Volandes to a patient and her husband who weren't much younger than me seemed needlessly distancing.

Lillian's husband lowered the volume on

the small speakers by her bedside and stood up, straightening his shirt collar. "This is Lillian, Angelo, and I am her husband, Raffi."

"Hi, Angelo," Lillian said, struggling to sit upright.

"Hi, Lillian. How are you feeling?" What a ridiculous thing to say to someone so clearly in pain.

"I'm okay." She immediately seemed to regret answering and trying to sit up, since the slightest movement wreaked havoc with her body, producing immediate pangs and spasms of intense pain.

"Meet our three beautiful boys, Angelo: Vartan, Aram, and our youngest, Raffi Junior." Raffi pointed to the previous year's Christmas photograph of himself and a much healthier-looking Lillian with the boys. "Merry Christmas from the Badakians" read the card. I could not help but note that the next family holiday picture would include one less Badakian.

"Angelo, is that Italian?"

"Actually, it's Greek."

"Greek, of course! Yasou! We have many Greeks in our Armenian church. Are you married?" I had many Armenian friends, and apart from language, the cultures had much in common: Life was deeply rooted in family traditions and revolved around the church and the community, and, most important, getting married and producing offspring.

"Married with one beautiful daughter."

"Our boys are two, four, and six," Lillian said proudly, a faint smile on her face. "They're why I keep going." Her pain had become intolerable, and she pushed the button on the patient-controlled medicine dispenser to receive another dose of morphine.

"We're hoping to be home for Easter dinner with the boys. Lillian wants to be home for Easter," Raffi added.

I counted the number of days until Easter; it was almost a month away. Did they really think Lillian would survive until Easter? I was not convinced that she would survive over the next few days, let alone a month from now.

"Lillian, what's your understanding of your disease, of how things are going?"

"Things aren't too good, not working as well as we hoped."

"Have you spoken with your oncologists and primary care doctors about what your options might be at this juncture?"

"We have focused on trying everything, anything. Raffi is always searching the Internet for something new," said Lillian, her words punctuated by long pauses as she fought back the pain.

"You never know what new chemo is on the way. There's always a chance we can cure this." Raffi's voice was both hopeful and desperate. It was no different from the many spouses and families I had met over the years: Professor Stone, Nonna's daughter Annunziata, Miguel's wife and daughter, Tom's wife and sister, and yes, even my own family. I thought of each one as Raffi confronted the impending death of his young wife.

There was little time to waste. Lillian was dying quickly. Choices needed to be made now about how she wanted to spend her remaining time in this world: in the hospital connected to IV poles with the slim hope of improvement and virtually no chance of recovery, or at home surrounded by her family. To make matters more complicated, there were three young children to consider. If Lillian died at the hospital, her children would be spared a final memory of their mother dying in the home they would continue to live in after her death. A decision needed to be made.

"There is always hope," I said, "but your cancer is very advanced and has spread to your bones. I want to communicate openly with both of you. Together, we can figure out what makes the most sense for you and your family, Lillian."

Was I being too forward, too honest? Still, I pushed on, determined that Lillian and Raffi should have all the facts they needed. "You have a choice, but I need to know what's important to you right now in your life. I need to understand what gives you meaning and fulfillment. We can continue all the medicines in the hospital and try to control your pain, understanding that your chances of recovery are very slim, or we can go another route and try to get you home or maybe into a nursing home so you can spend as much time as possible with your three boys. We would make sure you had the medicines you needed to control pain and someone to assist you."

I think they understood me, but I needed them to see what I was talking about. It would not be fair to Lillian, Raffi, or their boys if Lillian did not understand what her experience could be if she stayed in the hospital or went home, or perhaps to a nursing home. I placed a chair by her bedside, pulled an iPad from my coat pocket, and sat down. "Let's watch this short educational video together; it will review the same options but visually. I just want to make sure that we're all on the same page."

Raffi held the iPad and positioned it so that both he and Lillian could see the video that reviewed the goals of care for patients with a serious illness, the same video that I had shown Tom and his family as well as many other patients and their families, including my dad.

"This is incredibly helpful, Angelo," said Raffi, his eyes glued to the screen.

When it was over, I sensed that they wanted some privacy. "Why don't I step out for a few minutes? Go ahead and replay the video if you wish and discuss things together. I'll be back soon and we can continue the discussion."

As I walked back to the nurses' station, I pondered Lillian's predicament. She had three young boys at home, and her youngest, Raffi Jr., would only now be forming lasting images of his mother. Their one last Easter together — if she survived until then — might be the single memory that he would hold of his mother forever. And what if I were wrong? What if there was a miracle cure right around the corner? Not too long ago patients with melanoma were given the same grim news that I gave Lillian, and yet two recently discovered medicines can now offer these patients a few more months of life. For Lillian, that would allow Raffi Jr. to have more precious time with his mother.

Still, I knew the dismal statistics. Lillian's cancer was advanced despite every known therapy. I had seen many patients in the last stages of advanced terminal cancer just like Lillian, and every single one had died within weeks. When patients reach this point, there are no miracles, only false hopes and the reality of impending death. We needed to make the best of Lillian's situation. Did she imagine her death in the hospital or at home? Did she want her children with her at the end, or would that be too painful a memory for them? She was in so much pain; did we even have enough time to arrange the support she would need if she were to spend the rest of her days at home? There was much to consider. I returned to their room.

"Lillian and I want to thank you, Angelo, for helping us sort things out, especially with the video. I think we understand things perfectly. And I think that right now the best thing for our family is for Lillian to pursue life-prolonging care. If you can get us through one last Easter dinner together with the family, we can then revisit this decision."

"Lillian, is that what you want?"

"Yes."

I was not sure if the tears streaming down her cheeks were from the pain of the spreading cancer or from her predicament. Lillian would remain a full code. I gently hugged both of them and said I would honor their choice and support them through this.

At seven the next morning, my team met in the cafeteria to begin rounds. Although I was physically present during rounds, my mind was elsewhere. I could not stop thinking about Lillian, Raffi, and their boys. Lillian was going to die soon, and there was little that I could do. I thought of my own young daughter and what her life would be like if my wife or I died suddenly. Would she remember us? Doctors are reminded daily that it is simply a whim of fate that we are on the listening side of a stethoscope. "There, but for the grace of God, go I" is this doctor's daily prayer.

My thoughts were interrupted by the siren call of medical emergency: "Code Blue, Greenberg Five! Code Blue, Greenberg Five!"

We ran. Lillian was in trouble. We skipped the elevators — too slow — and hurried up the stairway.

Raffi was pacing in the hallway outside Lillian's room. We made brief eye contact as I entered. The nurses had already started CPR. I told my resident to take charge and run the code by the foot of Lillian's bed. "Please continue chest compressions and let's secure an airway. Get the heart monitor and pads ready in case we need to shock a V-fib arrest." She was a senior resident, one of the best. I trusted her to run the code on her own. Besides, I was needed elsewhere. I went out to speak to Lillian's husband.

"Raffi, Lillian's heart has stopped. We are performing CPR. Do you want to be with her?" When I was a resident a decade ago, this request would have been unheard of; families were never allowed to be present during a code. The fear was that the brutality of the procedure would be scarring and psychologically traumatic to loved ones. But as my medical school professor always told me, "Half of the things we teach you today will change by the time you practice medicine. We just don't know which half."

The presence of family members during resuscitation is no longer uncommon in hospitals. It usually occurs in emergency departments and occasionally in the ICU. Numerous studies conducted over the past decade have bolstered the practice, confirming that almost all family members who witness CPR performed on their loved ones say later that they would do so again. Seeing it done decreased their anxiety and fear about what was happening, facilitated their need to be together and support their loved one, and added a sense of closure that eased the grief process. Witnessing the procedure also removes any doubt that everything possible was done. And Raffi needed to know that he and Lillian had tried everything possible.

"I should be with her," Raffi said.

I took his arm and guided him into the room toward the head of Lillian's bed. One nurse was vigorously performing compressions on Lillian's chest, another was pumping air into her lungs with a green breathing bag, and another was administering lifesaving medications. No one skipped a beat as Raffi made his way to Lillian and bent toward her ear, whispering softly.

"Please stop compressions, and let's check for a pulse," my resident calmly instructed. There was no pulse. "Let's check the monitor. V-fib arrest. Please charge. Everybody clear the bed." Everyone, including Raffi, stepped back. "Shock. Check for a pulse. Resume compressions." Raffi continued to whisper softly in Lillian's ear.

As the senior physician, my function was

to make sure that what we were doing was the right thing, what the patient and her loved one felt was best for them. I stood behind Raffi, my hand on his shoulder, letting him know what we were doing during the code and encouraging him to keep speaking to Lillian.

I do not remember how long it lasted, what medicines we gave, or whether Lillian remained in ventricular fibrillation, but at some point, a point that felt right for Raffi, he asked us to stop. "Please stop. Thank you. My three little boys thank you for trying, for helping their mommy."

The nurses halted compressions and stopped pumping air into Lillian's lungs while one of the residents wiped away some of the blood that had seeped from the IVs. There was not a pair of dry eyes in the room. Most of us were more or less the same age as Lillian and Raffi, and many of us had young children. The team members filed out of the room so that Raffi could be alone with Lillian. I still had my hand on his shoulder and told him I was sorry that we could not do more.

"You did everything you could. We knew what the chances were and what might happen. We did the right thing for our boys. No regrets." He began to whisper softly into Lillian's ear, still tightly clasping her hand.

I looked at Lillian's face and then studied the photograph of the boys wearing their Santa hats. Each one resembled Lillian. How many holidays would go by before they would be happy again?

"Brooklyn Bridge!" my daughter called out from the backseat.

"And if Brooklyn has a bridge, shouldn't the other borough have one named after it, too?" I asked.

"Manhattan Bridge!"

"Good girl!"

My wife, our daughter, and I were driving down from Boston to New York City for Easter dinner with my father and mother. Our daughter was finally old enough to play the bridge game with me. I had tried playing the game with the names of Boston bridges, but somehow the Zakim and Long-fellow bridges didn't have the same magic. There was no nostalgia in hearing Boston bridges, and children's games are as much for parents as they are for children.

I could hear my father's voice echoing in the car. It had been years since I'd heard the booming voice only a child perceives, not his present voice, which had lost much of its husky timbre since his first heart attack. Had his voice ever really been that thunderous? It did not matter. It was his voice, as I remembered it.

This year's Easter dinner was going to be slightly different from previous ones. Mom's roast lamb, spanakopita, and endless rows of baklava would be on the table, but the table would be located in the rehabilitation facility's cafeteria. My father was doing well with his physical therapy, but not well enough to make it home by Easter. The one consolation was that at least he would eat food that reminded him of home instead of the unsalted food from the cafeteria.

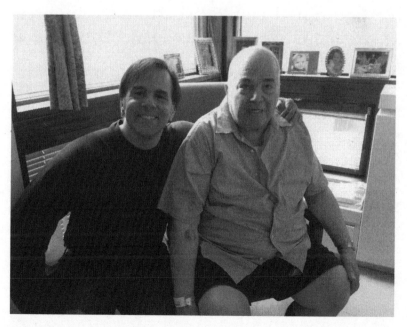

The author with his father at the rehabilitation facility.

I was slowly getting accustomed to the new normal. Dad would not likely be able to manage things at home the way he had. Taking out the trash, walking to the grocery store, helping my mother prepare the holiday dinners — he would need assistance with all of these activities.

I had to accept the change in his goals of medical care. One day in the future, I would likely get paged from a New York City number, perhaps from my mother or from a resident admitting my father to the hospital. I would be asked, as I always have been as the physician in the family, "Dr. Volandes, what is your father's code status?" And for the first time I would use those three letters in the same sentence as Dad. "My dad is DNR."

My parents had had The Conversation and had made a decision about the type of medical care they wanted, what made sense for them, and — from their perspective — for their family. They had the opportunity to consider the risks and benefits of many of the life-prolonging technologies that are available in today's hospitals, and realized there are limits to the latest and greatest that technology has to offer.

They also supplemented their discussions with their doctors with a video to ensure that they understood their choices and what each entailed. When patients have honest exchanges and have the tools necessary to understand their choices at the end of life, then they — not the health care system — remain in charge of decisions about how they want to live.

Making sure that patients have discussions early and often and receive the type of health care they desire at the end of life is the only way to rectify the appalling misalignment of the type of medical care that people receive at the end of life and the type of medical care they truly desire, whether it is a full code, comfort care, or something in between. The health care system must make sure that the type of medical care patients receive at the end of life is consistent with their preferences. "To deliver the right care, at the right time, and on the patient's terms" should be in the mission statement of all hospitals.

As I pulled the car into a New York City parking lot near my father's rehabilitation facility, my thoughts traveled a couple hundred miles north, back to Boston. In the Badakian home that Easter Sunday, three young boys were without their mother, likely confused by her premature death despite their father's attempts to console them. I hoped Raffi took some comfort in the fact that he and his wife had decided how they wished to spend the last few moments of her life, including the moment he chose to let her go.

As I opened the car door and unbuckled my daughter from the backseat, I lifted her up to my chest and vowed to do my part and continue The Conversation with all my patients.

AFTERWORD:
"NO ONE EVER ASKED ME
WHAT I WANTED"

At the ripe old age of eighty-nine, Mr. Tanaka had lived through two wars, the indignity of Japanese internment camps, a happy marriage to his wife of sixty years, the birth of five children, the death of his wife, and the scattering of dozens of grandchildren and great-grandchildren throughout the country. Now he was being shuffled between his nursing home and a large hospital in Honolulu.

Seeking a more relaxed life, Mr. Tanaka and his wife had decided to retire in Hawaii, so they sold their West Coast ranch house and bought a condo in Honolulu. Their life in tropical paradise was highlighted with Christmas visits with their children and the myriad visits by grandchildren and great-grandchildren during spring break. All of that changed after the death of his wife. Soon, Mr. Tanaka was no longer able to care for himself at home. He sold the condo and moved into an assisted living complex; in time, he graduated to the nursing home wing of the facility.

The slow winding down of his body brought with it urinary infections and other difficulties. With each complication, he was transferred to the hospital and then back to the nursing home. This happened so frequently that he often wondered why the hospital bothered sending him back. This time, once home, he would not return.

"Mr. Tanaka, we want to honor and respect your choices regarding medical care," a doctor from the nursing home told him. "We are starting a new statewide initiative by asking all of our residents for their thoughts. Have you ever had a discussion with your family about your wishes for medical care? About how you want to live your life?"

Mr. Tanaka shook his head.

"Well, it's never too late to start, even at eighty-nine. In order to get the discussion going, let's review this educational video that others have found to be really helpful. Would you prefer it in English or Japanese?"

Mr. Tanaka was surprised to be able to view the video in his native Japanese. He rarely had the opportunity to speak Japanese with his children, who preferred to speak

English, and he had all but given up on his grandchildren, who had no knowledge of the language. He indicated that he preferred the Japanese version and silently watched the video, carefully absorbing each word and image.

When the video ended, the doctor asked Mr. Tanaka if he had any thoughts. He paused and then responded.

"No one ever asked me what I wanted. I have lived for eighty-nine years in this country, and this is the first time that anyone has ever asked me what I want."

For the next few minutes, Mr. Tanaka and the doctor discussed the joy of smelling the fragrant Hawaiian plumeria in the nursing home's garden and the bliss of the morning sun warming his skin — the things that gave meaning to his life. He also expressed his wish to focus on the quality of each day that he had left, not the quantity. At the age of eighty-nine, with many medical decisions yet to be made, he was taking control of his medical care and his destiny.

Mr. Tanaka's is only one of many patient stories that are emerging from the state of Hawaii, an epicenter of health care innovation in improving the quality of care at the end of life. As part of a three-year project to transform its health system, the entire state is making The Conversation a priority. It is a massive effort led by the nonprofit Hawaii Medical Service Association, along with almost all of the hospitals, nursing homes, insurers, clinicians, and hospice facilities in the state — about a thousand different entities.

Residents of the state who are facing decision-making at the end of life are being encouraged to start discussions with their families and clinicians. To spark these exchanges and to empower people to understand their options, people have the opportunity to review a video with their doctors and nurses. The video has been translated into several languages spoken in the state. The goal of this monumental effort is to change the culture around this issue and to have patients "at the center of, in control of, and responsible for their own well-being."

On a day that I was visiting, one of the nurses I interviewed recounted a recent conversation with a patient. She had admitted an elderly man, originally from the Philippines, to the hospital for shortness of breath due to his advanced heart disease. She reviewed his history with him, his medications, any allergies he might have, and then began a discussion with him about his preferences for medical care.

As she pressed the "play" button on her tablet computer to view the video with him, he asked her, "Is that the video that goes over medical care and my three choices?" It turned out that he had watched a video in his primary care doctor's office, had started a discussion with his doctor, and even had completed documents indicating his wishes for medical care.

Many patients in Hawaii are having The Conversation after viewing the video as a result of the hard work of the consortium of providers and payers. Discussions are occurring in clinics, on hospital visits, and even at group meetings at nursing home communities like Mr. Tanaka's. Can we envision a day when clinicians slow down, no longer reflexively reach for the latest medical gadgets, and prioritize talking to patients?

Hawaii is one of the first states that have prioritized changing the culture of medical care, but it is not alone; other states are following Hawaii's example. In addition, enormous health care systems like Kaiser Permanente, large academic and small community hospitals, and clinics in urban and rural areas are dedicating themselves to changing the status quo by emphasizing the importance of having The Conversation with patients and families to make sure that they get the care they want and on their own terms.

As I traveled back to Boston from Hawaii, I reviewed a recent medical study that reminded me how far the health care system has to go before patients are at the center and in charge of their medical care. In this study, a group of patients with serious illness were admitted to a hospital and followed for one year. Prior to the study, many of these patients had not had The Conversation with their doctors.

At the study's outset, patients were asked about their preferences for medical care. About half preferred not to have invasive interventions like CPR or breathing machines. The patients were then followed for a year to see what happened to them over time. A fifth of those who stated that they did not want burdensome medical interventions received such care nonetheless. They were connected to breathing machines and underwent unwanted procedures. The reasons for the unwanted care included: missing or inaccurate documentation; miscommunication among providers; and, most important, doctors' failure to have The Conversation with patients. If doctors don't

214

engage patients and ask them their preferences for medical care, then patients will be defaulted to receiving all life-prolonging interventions — whether or not they desire them. In the end, unwanted medical care boils down to the foundational issue of informed consent. Patients with a serious illness often receive medical interventions for which they never gave consent. Worse yet, these medical errors are entirely preventable if doctors, nurses, and social workers have done their due diligence and engaged patients in these conversations.

Medical errors are usually described as human errors in which doctors choose an inappropriate intervention or method of care. Examples of medical errors include performing surgery on the wrong site, administering medication to the wrong patient, or giving the wrong blood type to a patient during a blood transfusion. Invasive medical interventions — like CPR, breathing machines, and feeding tubes — performed without a patient's consent must also be considered medical errors.

As the airplane began its descent into Boston, I stared out the window and reminded myself of all the unwanted care for which I had been personally responsible over the course of my career. There had been many times that I, too, had not stopped to have The Conversation, times when I had started a cascading series of medical procedures without ever asking the patient what he or she wanted. For physicians to start reprogramming themselves to ask what a patient wants before taking all possible steps to prolong that patient's life, they must first acknowledge the painful shortcomings from their past. This book has been my diary and confession about that experience.

My hope is that all people get the opportunity to live the way they wish, throughout all the chapters of their lives. Until that is achieved, I will continue to "strive in regards to disease two things, to do good or not to do harm."

APPENDIX I
STARTING THE
CONVERSATION
(FOR PATIENTS)

It has been many years since I first broached The Conversation with a patient. Since then, I have had hundreds of discussions with patients and families. My approach to these exchanges has changed over time; each dialogue has molded subsequent ones. Patients long since dead still live on in my discussions with new patients.

Although these exchanges are by no means easy, there is a common approach that can be learned. I encourage patients to start having these discussions early and often. The stories in my book are potent reminders of how wrong medical care can be at the end of life if patients fail to start the dialogue on their own.

LESSON #1: HAVE THE CONVERSATION

The moral of Taras Skripchenko's story: Don't wait for your doctor to start The

217

Conversation; start the discussion on your own with family members, friends, and your health care team.

Medical training focuses on the promise of medical technology, not communication skills; discussions about medical care consume a good deal of time in an otherwise short patient-doctor visit; and at present, there are few structural and financial supports to encourage doctors to start these exchanges. Patients should be prepared to start the process on their own.

Here are four important questions that can help you think about what is meaningful to you regarding medical care. I recommend that patients sit down with a pen and paper (or a laptop), answer these questions, and be sure to save the responses.

1. What kind of things are most important to you? What makes you happy?
At different stages in life, different things are important. For Tom Callahan, the most important thing in his life was being at home with family, as well as being able to sing his Irish songs. These activities gave Tom value and meaning in his life. For my parents, at this stage in their lives, being with their grandchildren and not burdening their children are most important to them,

and those considerations guide their decision-making.

2. What fears do you have about getting sick or needing medical care?

When I asked one of my patients this question, she looked at me and said, "I fear not being clean, dry, and intact. I also fear being in pain." Many people fear loss of independence due to illness. Nonna Bruno was no longer able to bathe herself, to feed herself, to think for herself, or to go to the bathroom on her own. For many, the fear of not being in control is overwhelming, and closely tied to the issue of control is the fear of being in intense pain and suffering. It is important to acknowledge your fears and concerns when having conversations about medical care at the end of life so that you can live in the here and now and plan for your future.

3. If you were very sick, are there any specific medical treatments that might be too much for you?

Some people find the thought of being in the advanced stages of illness and connected to a ventilator or life-support machines so dreadful that they would prefer never to experience it. Others feel that choosing such interventions reflects their will to live. For Professor Helen Thompson, seeing what breathing machines and life-prolonging interventions looked like while on her tour in the ICU was too much to bear; Miguel Sánchez experienced intubation to know that he never wanted it again. Lillian Badakian felt otherwise. How much medical care is enough for you? What is too much? What feels just right? This is a highly individualized decision and requires a significant amount of introspection.

If you aren't aware of the different types of treatments that are available to very sick people, now is the time to learn more.

4. Do you have any beliefs that guide you when you make medical decisions?

For many, spiritual, religious, philosophical, and cultural beliefs give order and meaning to their lives. Such beliefs may help guide decisions about medical care. For Nonna's family and for Tom's family, Catholicism and prayer were critical ingredients to understanding the toll disease was taking on their families. For Elijah Jones, he felt that God had given him additional time to live before calling him home. For others, philosophical and cultural beliefs may serve a similar role.

Considering these questions should not be a one-time event but rather a process you return to over time. The answers to these questions may change as your health status changes. For patients with significant illness, it might also be helpful to also think about four additional questions:

1. How do you value quantity versus quality of life? How important is it to you to live as long as possible, even if it means that you would experience pain and suffering?
2. If you had to choose between the length of life and the quality of life, which would be more important to you?
3. Is there a special occasion coming up that you would do anything to make sure you were present for?
4. Would you want to avoid pain at all costs even if you might not be able to interact with others?
5. How important is it to you to be at home when you die?

Lillian Badakian was willing to experience severe pain for the possibility of sharing one last holiday together as a family. For others, quality of life may be paramount, and avoiding pain and suffering are more primary considerations.

These are not easy questions, and it's normal to feel uncomfortable mulling them over. However, you can't afford not to make decisions.

LESSON #2: LET YOUR LOVED ONES KNOW YOUR CHOICES

The moral of Nonna Bruno's and Miguel Sánchez's stories: Don't keep your thoughts to yourself. Tell your loved ones your decisions about medical care before you sign and complete the appropriate paperwork.

When a patient is unable to make decisions for his or her medical care due to illness, doctors often look to the patient's spouse, family members, and friends for guidance. Unfortunately, many are unaware of what their loved ones would have wanted at the end of life. Sometimes family dynamics are such that family members make choices that the patient would never have agreed to, especially if the patient had been informed by his or her doctors of the options for medical care.

I often encourage patients to start the discussion with their loved ones during a holiday gathering. At the next family get-together, consider talking to your family about your choices. You do not need to establish everything with one conversation. It might take some time for your loved ones to feel comfortable talking about this subject. Start by picking a calm and quiet place to talk, maybe during a leisurely walk or a long drive.

Using a simple but direct icebreaker is a good way to start the discussion. You can refer to a relative or friend who passed away, cite a news article about illness, or even make a reference to the issue as it comes up in popular culture. Alternatively, you may consider sharing your concerns or beliefs about what makes your life worth living as a way to start the discussion. These conversations can be emotionally charged and your loved ones may initially be hesitant to talk, but assure them that having this discussion is very important to you. The talk does not need to have a certain structure; let it just happen. But make certain to emphasize points that are important to you.

Afterward, I encourage you to write a note or a letter about your discussion and share it with your family. Some people use their iPhone, iPad, or tablet to record their thoughts and wishes to video and to e-mail the recording to their loved ones. What do you want to remember about your talk? What are the next steps? If your family members or friends did not respond the way you wanted, try again later. It may take time for your loved ones to recognize that this is important to you.

Finally, and if you are ready, find out what documentation you need to fill out and complete. (See Appendix II for details about assigning your health care proxy and completing a living will.)

LESSON #3: TALK TO YOUR DOCTOR AND KNOW YOUR OPTIONS

The moral of Helen Thompson's and Elijah Jones's stories: Talk to your doctor. Know your options. Knowledge is power and in today's visually literate world, videos can help you better understand your options.

Once you have reflected on what's important to you (Lesson #1) and you have shared those thoughts with your family and friends (Lesson #2), it is time to translate those preferences into writing, which will require communication with your doctor (Lesson #3).

Many doctors will not raise the issue of end-of-life care, so you might have to be proactive. Let your doctor know that you are completing advance directives and share your thoughts about what in life is important to you. It can be as easy as saying "Dr. Volandes, I want to talk with you about my choices for medical care if I become seriously ill." Make sure that your doctor is willing to follow your instructions, and that he or she has copies on file or embedded in your electronic medical records.

Not enough patients inquire about a doctor's approach to medical treatments as it pertains to end-of-life care when choosing their physician. When selecting a potential health care provider, many patients ask where a doctor went to medical school, whether the doctor is male or female, young or old, and even whether the doctor has office hours on weekends. Although these may all be important factors in one's choice of physician, an equally important criterion for selecting your doctor is whether or not you can trust him or her to be honest with you when you have a serious illness. Will your doctor talk openly and honestly with you and your family if you have a serious illness? Will your doctor let you and your family know when treatments are no longer effective so that you can make choices that are consistent with your values? Will your doctor help you connect with experts in making sure that you are not in pain and have the support you need at the end of life? Having a doctor that you can trust during one of the most vulnerable periods in your life is far more important than your doctor's gender or age. When it comes to getting high-quality medical care that you want at the end of life, it's important that the two of you understand and agree with each other.

Speaking about your choices for medical care with your doctor is vital, since many of the key facts regarding your overall health will be known only to him or her. This is important when you make your decisions because the prognosis of a disease may determine which course of action you decide to take. Helen was suffering from a terminal, swiftly growing brain tumor. Elijah's kidneys were no longer functioning. The decisions that each of them made hinged on the terminal nature of their disease and their potential medical paths. Your doctor is the only person who can offer such details, and he or she is the only individual who can translate your wishes into an actionable medical plan.

Regardless of where you live or in which hospital you receive medical care, doctors will distinguish three conceptual categories called goals of care: **Life-Prolonging Care**, **Limited Medical Care**, and **Comfort Care**.

Life-Prolonging Care aims to prolong life at any cost. It translates into all potentially indicated medical care that is available in a modern-day hospital, including CPR, breathing machines, and treatment in the intensive care unit.

Limited Medical Care aims to maintain physical functioning and is consistent with treatments such as hospitalization, intravenous fluids, and medications, but not with CPR and invasive treatments in the medical intensive care unit.

Comfort Care aims to maximize comfort and to relieve pain. Only supportive measures that provide comfort are performed. It is compatible with oxygen and pain medications, but not with invasive therapies and hospitalization unless necessary to provide comfort.

Here is a link to a video that will review the three categories of medical care, as well as each of the three steps to Starting The Conversation so that you can be empowered to get the right care at the right time and on your terms.

http://www.theconversationbook.org

APPENDIX II
TAKING CONTROL AND COMPLETING YOUR ADVANCE DIRECTIVES

Over the course of your life, you have been able to make many important choices. Being able to make these choices has been a basic part of who you are as a person. Many of us take for granted that we will always be able to make our own decisions. But in life there are things that we may not be able to control — like getting sick. And sometimes, when people are very sick, they are not able to make decisions about medical care.

You might not be facing any serious medical issues right now. Maybe you haven't thought much about what might happen if you become very sick. But, in some ways, our health is a lot like the weather. You might not know that a storm is brewing or when it might hit. And once it hits, it's too late to get ready. Preparing would help you and your family weather the storm. That's why it's important to talk to your family and health care provider about the type of medical care you would want before the storm hits. These plans assure everyone that the care you receive would be the care that you want.

Advance directives are documents that can help make sure that you get the medical care that you desire. Below is a general guide to help you start thinking about advance directives and how you can remain in charge of your health care.

WHAT IS AN ADVANCE DIRECTIVE?

An advance directive is a legal document. It explains what type of medical care you would want in the event you are unable to speak for yourself. It also can say who would speak for you if this happened.

Advance directives generally come in two variants. A **living will** is a written document that explains what your wishes are for medical care. A **health care proxy** form says who you want to have the authority to make medical decisions for you. Sometimes, these documents are combined into one form. Although a living will can help reduce confusion about your treatment choices, it is still only a guide. It cannot predict every possible circumstance in which a medical decision may need to be made. Having an informed health care proxy can help make sure that your wishes are being honored. If you decide to have both documents, you should make sure that they do not conflict.

WHAT IS A LIVING WILL?

A living will is a document that explains what medical treatments you would want if you become very sick and are unable to speak for yourself. It may be called something else depending on what state you live in. It may be a standard form, and there are different kinds of living wills that you can download from the Internet.

For example, in a living will you can provide instructions about CPR, breathing machines, and other medical treatments. If you have any questions about what treatments you may or may not want, you should talk to your primary care doctor.

You do not need a lawyer to make a living will. There are, however, certain rules that must be followed to make the living will valid. If you feel that your wishes cannot be expressed to your satisfaction by a standard form, then you might want to have a lawyer help you create a document specifically for you.

It's important to understand that a living will is different from a will and testament. It does not deal with the handling of your finances or property. It deals only with medical issues while you are alive. A will and testament is for your estate. A living will is for medical decisions.

Here is a link provided by the Center to Advance Palliative Care that includes information and resources: www.getpalliativecare .org.

Each state has a different form that asks various questions. It is best to review your state's form with your health care provider. If you have additional questions, seek legal advice from a lawyer.

WHAT IS A HEALTH CARE PROXY?

The term "health care proxy" might have a different name in your state such as health care surrogate, health care agent, or durable power of attorney for health care.

Your health care proxy is your spokesperson and is designated on a health care proxy form, which both the patient and the proxy usually have to sign (some forms also include signatures for witnesses). He or she must follow your oral and written instructions. Your proxy can make medical decisions for you if you are too ill or injured to speak for yourself. You can also delegate decision-making to your proxy even if you are able to make your own decisions. Some people want their proxy to speak for them even when they still have the ability to speak for themselves.

Simply naming someone to be your health care proxy is not enough. It's important that the two of you have a real conversation about your values and priorities. Your health care proxy may have to make important medical decisions. Take the time to make sure that he or she is prepared. Your proxy deserves to understand and know what is important to you and how you think about the use of medical treatments at the end of life.

How Do I Choose a Health Care Proxy?

Here are three pointers to help you with picking your proxy.

1. Make Sure Your Health Care Proxy Understands Your Values and Wishes

It's important that you choose someone who will make decisions that you are comfortable with. Make sure that this person knows you well, understands what is important to you, and could handle the responsibility of making medical decisions for you. Take the time to talk about these sensitive issues. This may be uncomfortable at first, but it's important that your spokesperson be able to make decisions that honor you and your wishes.

2. Make Sure Your Health Care Proxy Will Act on Your Wishes

It's important to pick someone who will follow your wishes and is able to separate his or her own feelings from yours. You might find out that your health care proxy has different views about treatment choices. Ask him or her, "Will you be able to respect my wishes even if you may not agree with them?"

A health care proxy needs to be a strong advocate on your behalf. He or she may need to be persistent and forceful and ask questions in order to get the information needed to make decisions. Even though your proxy has the legal right to make decisions about your medical care, it might be difficult for him or her to do so if your family members are not in agreement. It is important that you ask your proxy whether he or she could handle a situation in which there might be conflicting opinions between loved ones and/or medical personnel. Make sure your proxy feels comfortable accepting this sort of responsibility.

3. Make Sure Your Health Care Proxy Is Available When You Need Him or Her

Although having a family member as a health care proxy is often a good choice, it is not always the best choice. A friend who knows you well and lives in the same city as you might be a better choice than a family member you see rarely or who lives far away. Pick someone who is close to you and who you can easily get in contact with to talk about your decisions.

Your wishes and values might change over time, especially after experiences in the hospital. It's important that your spokesperson be available to discuss these issues on a periodic basis and as often as you need to.

WHAT DO I DO WITH MY COMPLETED ADVANCE DIRECTIVES?

Your advance directives need to travel with you as you receive medical care in different settings. After you have completed a living will and/or health care proxy form, you should make several copies. Give a copy to your health care proxy, to your primary care provider, and to close family members. Keep the original in a safe place at home where it can be easily found, and make sure to let people know where it is located.

If you do not have any close family members or friends, it is important that you share your advance directives with your primary care provider. You should also find out if you can file your advance directives at your local hospital in case you are admitted there in the future. Give your health care team a copy of your advance directives so that they can include them as part of your medical record.

The recent development of online registries of advance directives may make accessing these documents easier in the future for patients, families, and health care providers. Although there are still concerns about the security and privacy of cloud-based services, being able to leverage technology in this fashion to help preserve patients' wishes is promising.

CAN I CHANGE MY ADVANCE DIRECTIVES?

You can cancel or change anything in your advance directives at any time for any reason. Different states have different rules about how to do this. Find out what is needed in your state to properly make changes.

The above guide can't possibly address all

of the different issues that might come up during these discussions, and it is not intended to be a substitute for professional medical advice, diagnosis, or treatment. If you have a specific question or problem, please talk to a medical or legal professional for guidance.

For more information, see the following online resource sponsored by the National Institutes of Health and the National Institute of Nursing Research: www.nihsenior health.gov/endoflife/planningforcare/01 .html

And remember, there are no right or wrong choices when it comes to advance directives, only choices that are right or wrong for you. Please take the time to start thinking about these issues now.

APPENDIX III
STARTING THE
CONVERSATION
(FOR FAMILIES)

"Disease may invade the bodies of patients, but the experience of illness devastates all those around them."

Decisions at the end of life for many patients with an advanced illness are made by family members or friends. Nonna Bruno's and Miguel Sánchez's families were left with the responsibility of deciding their respective end-of-life medical care. Over the course of a lifetime, you are likely to face a similar situation in which you are the decision-maker for a seriously ill loved one.

We can anticipate many decision points regarding medical care for advanced illnesses. Patients with advanced dementia will eventually face decisions regarding feeding tubes, aspirations, intubations, and CPR; the complications, trajectories, and potential treatments of the disease are all known. The same can be said of patients with most advanced illnesses such as cancer,

239

heart failure, kidney disease, and lung disease. Patients with advanced cancer and heart failure will eventually face the issue of if and when hospice is appropriate; for patients with kidney disease, dialysis or medical management is a predictable future option, as are breathing machines for patients with advanced lung disease. Family members and friends must start the process of engaging their loved ones with a serious illness in exploring what is important to them and what interventions are consistent with their beliefs and choices.

Ignorance is no longer acceptable, and guessing what your loved one prefers is unsatisfactory when you have opportunities to broach these topics when they are in the earlier stages of their illness.

For children of patients, I often advise them to broach The Conversation with a recent news article covering a controversy regarding medical care: "Mom, I read in the paper about a family that went to court about medical care for their mother. The children had never discussed with her what was important to her at the end of life, which led to disagreements among the children. I want to make sure that this never happens to us. Can we talk about this? Can I ask you some questions?"

For spouses of patients, I usually recommend to start with the death of a recent relative and how well (or not so well) the experience went. "I can't believe Uncle Benjamin passed away. He suffered until the very end. Poor Aunt Hannah was left to make all those decisions on her own, guessing most of the time what he would want. I can imagine all the guilt she felt making those decisions, pursuing all those interventions that made him suffer with little hope for recovery. Do you think the two of us can talk about what's important to you?"

The most important message that you can convey to your loved one is that you are willing to have The Conversation with him or her. Make it easy for him or her to open up to you about hopes, fears, and wishes for the course of his or her life. Start the discussion with some simple positive questions:

1. What brings you happiness each day?
2. What gets you out of bed in the morning?
3. What are you looking forward to?

These warm-up questions will naturally lead to more challenging questions:

1. What is most important to you if your time is limited?
2. What are the important things that you want your friends, family, and/or doctors to understand about your wishes for end-of-life care?
3. What fears do you have about getting sick or needing medical care?
4. Are there certain symptoms (such as severe nausea and pain) that are difficult but that you are willing to accept? Would any symptoms make life not worth living?

These are not easy questions to answer and it is important to acknowledge to your loved one that his or her answers may change over time. So make sure to give him or her enough time to think about what's important. You don't have to cover every topic in one discussion.

As the discussion winds down, make sure to review with your loved one what was discussed: "Mom, thanks for talking to me about this. I want to make sure that I heard you right, so tell me if I didn't, okay? You said . . ."

I always encourage families and friends to record these discussions using their iPhones, iPads, or tablets. There is nothing more reassuring when you are in the moment, making these emotionally fraught decisions in the ICU or in the hospital or at home, than to be able to view a short video that reminds you to honor and respect the wishes that your loved one reviewed with you. Watching a video in which you can see your loved one express choices and values that honor his or her life will reaffirm your commitment to providing medical care consistent with his or her wishes.

When your discussion ends, make sure to say thank you. "Thanks, Mom. Knowing what you would want takes a load off my shoulders." And always end with what's most important; make sure to say "I love you."

APPENDIX IV
ONLINE RESOURCES

Below are some suggested online resources to help you remain in control of your health care.

1. Get Palliative Care (www.getpalliativecare .org)

No single individual has done more to improve the quality of care for patients than Dr. Diane Meier. For decades, Dr. Meier has been at the forefront of protecting the rights of patients at all stages in their lives. She created the Center to Advance Palliative Care (CAPC), which is a national organization dedicated to increasing the availability of quality services for people facing serious, complex illness. CAPC has created the Get Palliative Care Web site to better inform people about their options for medical care throughout the life-span, with or without a life-limiting condition.

2. The Conversation Project (www.thecon versationproject.org)

In 2010, the journalist Ellen Goodman began the Conversation Project. Ellen, along with a group of colleagues and concerned media, clergy, and medical professionals, gathered to share stories about personal experiences with end-of-life care. Since then, her work has blossomed into a national discussion about improving the quality of care at the end of life and encouraging everyone to have a dialogue with family members and friends. Ellen is a passionate advocate whose personal experience with caring for a sick family member has inspired thousands of others to take control of their lives. The Web site offers many resources to get started and share your thoughts with others.

3. PREPARE (www.prepareforyourcare .org)

PREPARE is a state-of-the-art online video program that assists patients and families in thinking about what is important to them about their medical care. It was developed by the incomparable Dr. Rebecca Sudore, a national leader in geriatrics who teaches at the University of California, San

Francisco. The interactive program includes videos and written tools to help individuals evaluate how to make decisions about medical care at the end of life.

None of the above Web sites is meant to replace a discussion with a professional medical provider. I would recommend starting with any of the three Web sites (why not all three!) and then set up an appointment with your health care provider to continue the dialogue.

ACKNOWLEDGMENTS

This book is not only an exploration of life's final chapter, but also a chronicle of my coming-of-age as a doctor. My guides along this journey remain the same teachers who have taught every physician: patients. These are their stories. I am profoundly indebted to each of them.

As a first-time author, I have had the good fortune to work with an amazing literary agent, editor, and publishing house. Will Lippincott, of Lippincott Massie McQuilkin, saw the early promise of this project and then shepherded it from start to finish. My editor, Nancy Miller, of Bloomsbury Publishing, provided invaluable editorial guidance, support, and encouragement. I am grateful to both of them for believing in this project.

Writing a book is a process, and one that rivals the grueling days and nights of training to be a physician. There were many readers of this manuscript who helped guide me along the way. I am especially thankful to Muriel Gillick, who helped me find my voice. I am also obliged to my inner circle of readers who have accompanied me on this journey: Elmer Abbo, Michael Paasche-Orlow, Hacho Bohossian, William Kennedy, and Areej El-Jawahri. I am especially thankful to Matt Handley, Elizabeth Marshall, Jonathan Rauch, Daniel Matlock, Robert J. Levine, Tia Powell, Lenny López, Sara Paasche-Orlow, and Jenn Shin, who read earlier versions of this book.

I owe a great debt to Professor Kirsty Milne for challenging me throughout the writing of this book on what it means to be on the other side of the stethoscope; I only wish she had lived to see it in print.

I am fortunate to lead a phenomenal group of innovative researchers. The Video Images of Disease for Ethical Outcomes (VIDEO) Consortium consists of many individuals from academic medical centers across the country. Their commitment and dedication to educating the public and increasing discussions between doctors and patients is unrivaled. I especially want to thank Michael Barry, Susan Mitchell, Elizabeth Walker-Corkery, Zara Cooper, Jennifer Temel, Vicki Anne Jackson, Josh Metlay,

Katrina Armstrong, Tom Smith, Andrew Epstein, Jane Schell, Ruth Carroll, Eileen Mann, Yuchiao Chang, Nwamaka Eneanya, Ann O'Hare, Alvin "Woody" Moss, Michael Germain, Manjula Tamura, Vincent Mor, JoanTeno, Lewis Cohen, Ariela Noy, Tomer Levin, Pat Agre, Fatima Rodriguez, Sam Rodriguez, Kenneth Minaker, Monera Wong, Ardeshir Hashmi, and Rebecca Aslakson for their unwavering support. A special thank-you goes to Diane Meier, who taught me the power of effecting change with patient stories.

I am also thankful to Hilton Raethel, Rae Seitz, Robert Eubanks, Lori Protzman, Michelle Cantillo, Daniel Fischberg, Anna Loengard, and the wonderful people of Hawaii for helping me translate this work into clinical practice in an effort to transform health care. I believe that the experience of Hawaii, "the little mouse that roars," will help improve the quality of care delivered to all Americans.

I am grateful to the Melik-Baschkopf Foundation and its directors, Edward H. Dietrich, Andrea Reiff, and Milton Kahn, for their financial support that continues to help change the culture of medicine around the country.

Three individuals who have raised awareness of The Conversation in the wider community include three giants in the field: Ellen Goodman, Bernard "Bud" Hammes, and Susan Tolle. Ellen has made honoring people's choices a social movement with the Conversation Project; Bud had a vision that has literally transformed the lives of thousands of Americans already with Respecting Choices; and Susan Tolle had the courage to preserve patients' voices when no one else did with the POLST paradigm. I am grateful to each one of them, and my work is a testament to their enduring influence on all of us.

With respect to the video, all of the medical staff, patients, and/or their families have permitted me to use their images and voices for the purposes of educating the public. Unlike names and facts that can be easily altered to protect confidentiality, visual images are far less malleable without distracting from their educational purpose. As such, for the most part I have not obscured the faces of the people in the videos. I am eternally grateful to the staff, patients, and families for their charitable gift to us all, and I strongly encourage my readers to consider and respect their gift.

My family of readers has helped me balance work, life, and writing during the decade it has taken me to craft this book. I am thankful to Peter Volandes, Ava Volandes, Sophia Volandes, Stellene Volandes, Cayla Volandes, Kenneth Volandes, Marina Volandes, Aleko Tavantzis, Angelos Konstas, Shane Genakos, Bennett Ruiz, and Jake Young.

A heartfelt thank-you to my loving mother-in-law, Winifred Maggie Davis, who, through her own personal struggles with end-of-life decision-making for her husband, my late wonderful father-in-law, informs many of these pages.

My parents deserve special thanks. Their experiences of coming to this country, not speaking a word of English, and toiling for years washing dishes and collecting nickel and dime tips in a New York City diner to help send their children to the best schools in the world is humbling. Thank you for giving me the Ancient Greek literature, poetry, drama, and philosophy books during childhood, when we could afford only the tattered, secondhand copies from the Salvation Army store. I love you both dearly, and the greatest gift I can give back to you is to introduce those same books and ideas to your grandchildren.

Most of all, I want to thank my wife, Aretha Delight Davis, and our two children,

Angeliki Agape and Evangelia Faith. From the second week of freshman year in college when we met, Aretha has remained my soul's perfect reflection. She has been my lifelong interlocutor and partner who, despite my imperfections, continues to tolerate my crazy ideas, like using our living room as a film studio. As an accomplished physician and lawyer in her own right, Aretha shaped my understanding of the practice of medicine at a systems level. Every word in this book has been influenced and molded by our endless conversations, a veritable Socratic dialogue in our living room. Thank you for remaining by my side and guiding me on this amazing writing journey and on our own journey together called life. Most of all, thank you for giving us the two greatest gifts in the world, our daughters. This book would not be possible without your love.

NOTES

I have taken the liberty of including the latest references to publications to support the medical points cited, even if those publications had not been carried out and/or published at the time of the events narrated. I felt it important to offer the reader the latest in terms of research publications. The medical events recounted in the narratives and included in this book are as accurate as I remember them, but medicine does change. The references included in these notes are for the reader's use if he or she wishes to explore the latest medical developments.

Introduction

"When asked where and how they want to spend their last few months, nearly 80 percent of Americans respond that they want to be at home with family

and friends, free from the institutional grip of hospitals and nursing homes, and in relative comfort." Many medical researchers have spent their careers documenting the preferences of patients regarding where they wish to receive medical care at the end of life. The research suggests that most people wish to die at home, in comfort, and surrounded by their loved ones. See: George H. Gallup International Institute. *Spiritual Beliefs and the Dying Process: A Report on a National Survey.* Conducted for the Nathan Cummings Foundation and the Fetzer Institute, 1997; Terri R. Fried et al. "Older Persons' Preferences for Site of Terminal Care." *Annals of Internal Medicine* 131, no. 2 (1999): 109–12; Kevin Brazil et al. "Preferences for Place of Care and Place of Death Among Informal Caregivers for the Terminally Ill." *Palliative Medicine* 19, no. 6 (2005): 492–99; and Andrea Gruneir et al. "Where People Die: A Multilevel Approach to Understanding Influences on Site of Death in America." *Medical Care Research and Review* 64, no. 4 (2007): 351–78.

"However, only 24 percent of Americans over sixty-five die at home; 63 percent die in hospitals or nursing homes,

sometimes tethered to machines, and often in pain." See: National Center for Health Statistics. *Health, United States, 2010: With Special Feature on Death and Dying.* http://www.cdc.gov/nchs/data/hus/hus10.pdf. Accessed June 14, 2014. Interestingly, data comparing place of death in 1989 as opposed to 2007 showed one important change. There was an increase in the number of people dying at home. For people over the age of sixty-five, in 1989, 15 percent of people died at home; in 2007 that number increased to 24 percent. However, an analysis of data during that same time period showed a more frightening observation: The rate of medical interventions and overall intensive care use in the last month of life increased, with about a third of people over sixty-five experiencing an intensive care unit hospitalization in the last months of life. An additional finding was that a large number of people over sixty-five had three or more hospitalizations in the last months of life. These findings by Dr. Joan Teno, who has dedicated her life to improving medical care for patients, rattled many in health care, showing as they do that despite a slight increase in the number of people dying at home, people are dying with more frequent visits to intensive care units and hospitals. See: Joan M. Teno et al. "Change in End-of-Life Care for Medicare Beneficiaries: Site of Death, Place of Care, and Health Care Transitions in 2000, 2005, and 2009." *Journal of the American Medical Association* 309, no. 5 (2013): 470–77. Also see the commentary in the same issue by Grace Jenq and Mary E. Tinetti. "Changes in End-of-Life Care over the Past Decade: More not Better." *Journal of the American Medical Association* 309, no. 5 (2013): 489–90. doi:10.1001/jama.2013 .73.

"Over the last few decades, clinicians who are experts in navigating hospitals and complex medical interventions have emerged." See National Hospice and Palliative Care Organization. "NHPCO Facts and Figures: Hospice Care in America." http://www.nhpco.org/ sites/default/files/public/Statistics_Re search/2011_Facts_Figures.pdf. Accessed June 14, 2014.

"These professionals usually reside in departments of palliative care." It is worth noting early on that I do not want to confuse palliative care with hospice care. The two are very different. Although both palliative and hospice care share the same philosophy by focusing on quality of life ("comfort care") and managing pain and the psychological and spiritual issues experienced at the end of life, they are different. Presently, hospice care is a Medicare benefit for patients who, to a doctor's best determination, have less than six months to live and who wish to forgo attempts at curative treatments. Palliative care does not depend on life expectancy and these services can be used throughout the life cycle. Palliative care focuses on improving the understanding of choices and provides communication support as well as emotional support for patients and families. I often involve palliative care services as soon as a diagnosis is made, regardless of life expectancy. My good friend Dr. Diane Meier probably said it best: "Hospice is a form of palliative care for people who are dying, but palliative care is not about dying. It's about living as well as you can for as long as you can." As the director of the Center to Advance Palliative Care, Diane lectures tirelessly about this distinction. See the interview with her in: Jane E. Brody. "Palliative Care, the Treatment That Respects Pain." *New York Times,* December 2, 2013. http://www.well.blogs.nytimes.com/2013/12/02/

palliative-care-the-treatment-that-respects
-pain/?_r=1. Accessed June 14, 2014.

"Patients pay the price for this short-sightedness and lack of funding, and in order to address the scale of the problem, all doctors, not just palliative care doctors, should be highly trained communicators who insist on discussions with patients about medical care at the end of life." The argument for expecting all clinicians to have the skills needed to be good communicators regarding care at the end of life was recently made by two giants in the field of medicine, Timothy Quill and Amy Abernethy. Both were recently named "top thirty visionaries of all time" by the American Academy of Hospice and Palliative Medicine (http://www.aahpm.org/about/default/visionaries.html). See: Timothy E. Quill and Amy P. Abernethy. "Generalist Plus Specialist Palliative Care: Creating a More Sustainable Model." *New England Journal of Medicine* 368, no. 13 (2013): 1173–75.

"The success of this essential conversation about end-of-life care lies not in the individual path chosen but rather in the active and fully informed participation of the patient and family

members." When physicians talk with patients and families about medical care at the end of life, they refer to these discussions as having "The Conversation." Although physicians have many different types of conversations with patients throughout the continuum of the life cycle, when using a capital *T* and *C*, physicians typically mean a discussion about end-of-life care. In other words, The Conversation of all conversations: talking about life-and-death decisions. The Conversation does not have to only occur between doctors and patients. The journalist Ellen Goodman has made a remarkable contribution to medicine by encouraging patients to have conversations with their loved ones outside of the medical setting with her innovative Conversation Project, which motivates people to talk about their choices for medical care at the end of life. In addition to Ellen, a group of innovators have created Death Over Dinner, a movement to encourage people to openly discuss their preferences for end-of-life care. One of the lead doctors in this movement is the masterful Dr. Anthony "Tony" Back, who has trained legions of clinicians to have The Conversation with their patients. See: Anthony Back et al. *Mastering Com-*

munication with Seriously Ill Patients: Balancing Honesty with Empathy and Hope (Cambridge: Cambridge University Press, 2009). In addition to Ellen and Tony, the dynamic Bernard "Bud" Hammes and the Respecting Choices program have trained clinicians and health care systems on improving the quality of discussions between doctors and patients. See: Kristen E. Pecanac et al. "Respecting Choices and Advance Directives in a Diverse Community." *Journal of Palliative Medicine* December 10, 2013. doi: 10.1089/jpm.2013.0047.

"In the case of those people who did not have the benefit of discussing their options, the stories of their end-of-life care exhibit the neglect that deeply permeates the U.S. health care system." Even with patients who have a terminal illness, doctors often do not have discussions about end-of-life care. See: Areej El-Jawahri et al. "Associations Among Prognostic Understanding, Quality of Life, and Mood in Patients with Advanced Cancer." *Cancer* 120, no. 2 (2014). doi: 10.1002/cncr.28369. Epub October 10, 2013, ahead of print.

"We answered the call of medicine in order to do good, yet the overwhelm-

ing majority of us treat patients with serious illness in a manner we would never want for our loved ones, or even for ourselves." What doctors would want at the end of life has been studied carefully, and for good reason. One of the most powerful predictors of what a patient decides regarding medical care is a physician's answer to the question "Doctor, what would you choose if you were in my shoes?" In one oft-cited study of physicians, 85 percent of physicians would forgo CPR and mechanical ventilation if they had a terminal brain injury. See: Joseph J. Gallo et al. "Life-Sustaining Treatments: What Do Physicians Want and Do They Express Their Wishes to Others?" *Journal of the American Geriatrics Society* 51, no. 7 (2003): 961–69. Also see: Gregory P. Gramelspacher et al. "Preferences of Physicians and Their Patients for End-of-Life Care." *Journal of General Internal Medicine* 12, no. 6 (1997): 346–51; and Garrett M. Chinn et al. "Physicians' Preferences for Hospice If They Were Terminally Ill and the Timing of Hospice Discussions with Their Patients." *JAMA Internal Medicine* 2014. doi:10.1001/jamainternmed.2013.12825.

"**Even today, some oncologists are hesitant to discuss medical care with patients in the advanced stages of cancer out of fear that they will dash any hope the patient clings to, despite the extensive medical research that indicates many patients do, in fact, want to talk about these topics with their physicians.**" See: Alexi A. Wright et al. "Associations Between End-of-Life Discussions, Patient Mental Health, Medical Care Near Death, and Caregiver Bereavement Adjustment." *Journal of the American Medical Association* 300, no. 14 (2008): 1665–73. doi: 10.1001/jama.300.14.1665. Also see: Peter A. Singer et al. "Quality End-of-Life Care: Patients' Perspectives." *Journal of the American Medical Association* 281, no. 2 (1999): 163–68; and Terri R. Fried and John R. O'Leary. "Using the Experiences of Bereaved Caregivers to Inform Patient- and Caregiver-Centered Advance Care Planning." *Journal of General Internal Medicine* 23, no. 10 (2008): 1602–07.

"**As far as the medical team was concerned, Taras was a 'full code,' because he had not requested a Do Not Resus-**

citate (DNR) order." The default for all patients regardless of their health is a "full code"; in other words, everything is presumed to be desired unless there are indications that the patient preferred otherwise. This default has come under intense scrutiny, especially in patients with advanced illness. See: Angelo E. Volandes and Elmer D. Abbo. "Flipping the Default: A Novel Approach to Cardiopulmonary Resuscitation in End-Stage Dementia." *Journal of Clinical Ethics* 18, no. 2 (2007): 122–39; Scott D. Halpern et al. "Default Options in Advanced Directives Influence How Patients Set Goals for End-of-Life Care." *Health Affairs* 32, no. 2 (2013): 408–17. doi: 10.1377/hlthaff.2012.0895; Caroline M. Quill et al. "Deciphering the Appropriateness of Defaults: The Need for Domain-Specific Evidence." *Journal of Medical Ethics* 38, no. 12 (2012): 721–22. doi: 10.1136/medethics-2012-100724; and Scott D. Halpern et al. "Harnessing the Power of Default Options to Improve Health Care." *New England Journal of Medicine* 357, no. 13 (2007):1340–44.

"In Rochester, medical students are assigned seriously ill patients from primary care clinics early in their training." See: Timothy E. Quill et al. "An

Integrated Biopsychosocial Approach to Palliative Care Training of Medical Students." *Journal of Palliative Medicine* 6, no. 3 (2003): 365–80.

"Dr. Meier describes such real student-patient interactions as 'the difference between watching a movie about war and being in war.' " https://www.aamc.org/newsroom/reporter/july2012/297224/palliative-care.html. Accessed June 14, 2014.

"In 2008, a group of Dartmouth researchers surveyed all 128 medical schools in the United States regarding offerings in 'Palliative and Hospice Care.' " See: Emily S. Van Aalst-Cohen et al. "Palliative Care in Medical School Curricula: A Survey of United States Medical Schools." *Journal of Palliative Medicine* 11, no. 9 (2008): 1200–2.

"Concurrent with the explosion of medical knowledge is the fact that residents are now limited to no more than eighty hours per week, which still constitutes a brutal workweek." I completed my medical residency more than a decade ago. It was not unusual for the medical residents to work more than one hundred hours per week; many of us slept at the hospital even if we were not the overnight physician. Since residency, a growing consensus among educators has recognized that long hours for residents lead to a sharp rise in medical errors due to sleep deprivation. The Accreditation Council for Graduate Medical Education has since limited the number of hours that a resident can work to eighty hours per week. Unfortunately, even eighty hours per week may still be too much (that's the equivalent of working two full-time jobs!). It remains to be seen if the eighty hours will be chiseled down further. See: Christopher P. Landrigan et al. "Effect of Reducing Interns' Work Hours on Serious Medical Errors in Intensive Care Units." *New England Journal of Medicine* 351, no. 18 (2004): 1838–48.

Chapter 2

"About a fifth of the patients admitted to the hospital have some form of dementia, a medical term encompassing various disorders associated with loss of memory and other cognitive difficulties that are severe enough to impede a person's ability to function in daily life." See: https://www.alz.org/

what-is-dementia.asp. Accessed June 14, 2014.

"In 2012, there were more than 35 million people in the world living with dementia . . ." See: http://www.who.int/mediacentre/factsheets/fs362/en. Accessed June 14, 2014. Also see: Ron Brookmeyer et al. "Projections of Alzheimer's Disease in the United States and the Public Health Impact of Delaying Disease Onset." *American Journal of Public Health* 88, no. 9 (1998): 1337–42; and Ron Brookmeyer et al. "Forecasting the Global Burden of Alzheimer's Disease." *Alzheimer's & Dementia* 3, no. 3 (2007): 186–91.

"The German psychiatrist Alois Alzheimer identified the first case of what would later be known as Alzheimer's disease more than a century ago, yet the disease remains 100 percent incurable and ultimately 100 percent fatal." For a thorough overview of Alzheimer's disease see Muriel Gillick's classic book *Tangled Minds: Alzheimer's Disease and Other Dementias.* (Cambridge: Harvard University Press, 1999).

"Equally problematic are misperceptions about the stages of Alzheimer's disease." I am indebted to Muriel Gillick for the many conversations we have had about the stages of Alzheimer's disease. With her permission, I have used many of her examples for the different stages of the disease as well as the overall conceptual framing of the stages.

"What kills you in the end is not Alzheimer's disease, but the consequences of the associated bodily deterioration as the mind shrivels: an infection in the urine, for example; or food trapped in the lungs; or a wound to the buttocks that has developed from immobility." The nationally recognized leader on the clinical course of advanced Alzheimer's disease is my mentor and frequent collaborator, Dr. Susan L. Mitchell. Susan has dedicated her life to improving the understanding of Alzheimer's disease and has published widely on this topic. See: Susan L. Mitchell et al. "The Clinical Course of Advanced Dementia." *New England Journal of Medicine* 361 (2009): 1529–38.

"Many people with advanced Alzheimer's disease require more care than their families can provide . . ." To get the family's perspective on caring for patients with Alzheimer's disease, the recommended book is by Nancy Mace and Peter Rabins, *The 36-Hour Day: A*

Family Guide to Caring for Persons with Alzheimer's Disease, Related Dementias, and Memory Loss in Later Life. (New York: Grand Central Life & Style, 2012).

"Medical evidence suggests that feeding tubes do not prolong survival in those patients." A large body of evidence suggests that feeding tubes are not helpful in advanced dementia. See: Susan L. Mitchell et al. "The Risk Factors and Impact on Survival of Feeding Tubes in Nursing Home Residents with Severely Advanced Dementia." *Archives of Internal Medicine* 157, no. 3 (1997): 327–32; Thomas E. Finucane et al. "Tube Feeding in Patients with Advanced Dementia: A Review of the Evidence." *Journal of the American Medical Association* 282, no. 14 (1999): 1365–70; Muriel R. Gillick. "Rethinking the Role of Tube Feeding in Patients with Advanced Dementia." *New England Journal of Medicine* 342 (2000): 206–10; and Muriel R. Gillick and Angelo E. Volandes. "The Standard of Caring: Why Do We Still Use Feeding Tubes in Patients with Advanced Dementia?" *Journal of the American Medical Directors Association* 9, no. 5 (2008): 364–67.

"In 2010, the *British Medical Journal* pub-

lished an article that followed families of seriously ill patients." See: Karen M. Detering et al. "The Impact of Advance Care Planning on End of Life Care in Elderly Patients: Randomised Controlled Trial." *British Medical Journal* 340 (2010): c1345.

"Nonna had designated a family member to assist in decision-making when she was no longer able to speak for herself." It is interesting to note that some cultures defer medical decisions to families when patients are no longer able to make decisions. This is particularly true in cultures in which the perspective of the community trumps individual autonomy. Designating a proxy is consistent with this framework, since a proxy can express such a view when the patient cannot speak for herself. It is also important to note that even if a medical decision is deferred to the family, in some cases family members hold conflicting opinions and one individual — the proxy — must ultimately decide for the patient. For more on cross-cultural considerations in medicine, see: Judy Ann Bigby, ed., *Cross-Cultural Medicine.* (Philadelphia: American College of Physicians, 2001).

"In 2006, researchers at the National Institutes of Health published one of the largest studies to look at the accuracy of health care proxy decisions." See: David I. Shalowitz et al. "The Accuracy of Surrogate Decision Makers: A Systematic Review." *Archives of Internal Medicine* 166, no. 5 (2006): 93–97.

"Living wills should not be confused with POLST (Physician Orders for Life-Sustaining Treatment) or MOLST (Medical Orders for Life-Sustaining Treatment) forms." See: http://www.polst.org. A good deal of the work done on POLST has been spearheaded by Dr. Susan Tolle, who revolutionized the practice of medicine with the POLST paradigm.

"A 2010 study published in the *New England Journal of Medicine* by researchers at the University of Michigan supports the use of living wills." See: Maria J. Silveira et al. "Advance Directives and Outcomes of Surrogate Decision Making Before Death." *New England Journal of Medicine* 362, no. 13 (2010): 1211–18.

"Although living wills were developed as a way to help people retain control of their medical care, in reality they have not met their promise." See: Angela Fagerlin and Carl E. Schneider. "Enough: The Failure of the Living Will." *Hastings Center Report* 34, no. 2 (2004): 30–42.

"Living wills are not always readily available to doctors when they need to review the forms; they can be too vague ('If I am close to death . . .') or too specific ('If I am in a permanent coma . . .') and can be open to subjective interpretation; and they frequently need to be revisited over time as a patient's health status changes." See: Hastings Center, "Improving End-of-Life Care: Why Has It Been So Difficult?" Hastings Center Report December 2005: 26–31.

"[Several major medical organizations] have promoted guidelines suggesting that physicians should have conversations about medical care for Alzheimer's disease in all patients over the age of sixty-five irrespective of whether they have been diagnosed with the illness." See the Society of General Internal Medicine (http://www.sgim.org), the American Geriatrics Society (http://www.americangeriatrics

.org), and the Gerontological Society of America (http://www.geron.org). The medical establishment considers preferences stated at the time prior to losing one's reasoning capacity as the preferences that ought to be respected throughout the life of a person. Philosophers, however, have raised some interesting issues surrounding personal identity and whether the preferences of previous selves should be preserved. If that sounds confusing, prepare to be more confused by reading the brilliant but inscrutable *Reasons and Persons* (1984) by Derek Parfit. I consider myself fortunate to have attended one of his classes in college where he presented some of the issues surrounding Alzheimer's disease and other personal identity conundrums. I am still trying to work them out in my mind decades later.

Chapter 3

"The American Heart Association estimates that there are more than five million people in the United States with heart failure." See: A. S. Go. "Heart Disease and Stroke Statistics 2013 Update: A Report from the American Heart Association." *Circulation* 127, no. 1

(2013): e6.

"Heart failure is the leading cause of hospitalization in people over sixty-five years of age." See: Akshay S. Desai and Lynne W. Stevenson. "Rehospitalization for Heart Failure: Predict or Prevent?" *Circulation* 126 (2012): 501–06.

"In 1991, a group of geriatricians published an article in the *Journal of the American Geriatrics Society* entitled 'Decision Making in the Incompetent Elderly: "The Daughter from California Syndrome." ' " See: D.W. Molloy et al. "Decision Making in the Incompetent Elderly: 'The Daughter from California Syndrome.' " *Journal of the American Geriatrics Society* 39, no. 4 (1991): 396–99.

"In California, this is known as the Daughter from New York Syndrome." See: Maurice D. Steinberg and Stuart J. Youngner, eds. *End-of-Life Decisions: A Psychosocial Perspective.* (Washington, D.C.: American Psychiatric Press, 1998), 92.

Chapter 4

"They're in the hospital for urgent care, and more often than not, their

doctors have not previously broached the issue of end-of-life care." Unfortunately, most doctors do not address end-of-life decision-making with patients until they are critically ill. There are many hypotheses as to why doctors do not broach these topics with patients early in the course of an illness. See: R. Sean Morrison et al. "Physician Reluctance to Discuss Advance Directives: An Empiric Investigation of Potential Barriers." *Archives of Internal Medicine* 154, no. 20 (1994): 2311–18. Also see: The SUPPORT Investigators. "A Controlled Trial to Improve Care for Seriously Ill Hospitalized Patients. The Study to Understand Prognoses and Preferences for Outcomes and Risks of Treatments (SUPPORT)." *Journal of the American Medical Association* 274 (1995): 1591–98.

"At the dawn of the twentieth century, William Osler, often referred to as the father of modern medicine, told a graduating class of medical students . . ." See: William Osler. "Aequanimitas." In *Aequanimitas with Other Addresses.* (Philadelphia: P. Blakiston's Son & Co., 1904), 7.

"Although doctors have a clearer sense of the prognosis when looking at the

big picture for certain illnesses, there will always be some degree of uncertainty in medicine, and it is hard to be content with finding broken portions." There is a fair amount of research around prognosis and physicians' ability to prognosticate patients' overall survival. See Nicholas Christakis, *Death Foretold: Prophecy and Prognosis in Medical Care* (University of Chicago Press, 2001). However, it is much more difficult to determine the timing of death (days versus weeks versus months) as the end of life nears. A good deal of uncertainty will always be present at the end of life. See also: Leah R. Evans et al. "Surrogate Decision-Makers' Perspectives on Discussing Prognosis in the Face of Uncertainty." *American Journal of Respiratory and Critical Care Medicine* 179, no. 2 (2009): 48–53; Lindsey C. Yourman et al. "Prognostic Indices for Older Adults: A Systematic Review." *Journal of the American Medical Association* 307, no. 2 (2012): 182–92; George Loewenstein. "Hot-Cold Empathy Gaps and Medical Decision Making." *Health Psychology* 24, no. 4 (2005): S49–S56; and, Nicholas A. Christakis and Elizabeth B. Lamont. "Extent and Determinants of Error in

Doctors' Prognoses in Terminally Ill Patients: Prospective Cohort Study." *British Medical Journal* 320 (2000): 469–72.

"It's called Cushing's Triad." When there is an increase in intracranial pressure, a series of physiological responses occur including a rise in blood pressure, an irregular breathing pattern, and a decrease in the heart rate. This physiological response is known as the Cushing reflex or Cushing's Law, named after the neurosurgeon Dr. Harvey Cushing, who first described this phenomenon in 1901. See: Harvey W. Cushing. "Concerning a Definite Regulatory Mechanism of the Vasomotor Center which Controls Blood Pressure During Cerebral Compression." *Bulletin of the Johns Hopkins Hospital* 126 (1901): 289–92.

"No large, well-conducted, scientific study has ever shown a significant association between personality traits and survival from cancer, but my guess is that no number of negative studies will ever extinguish this deeply held belief." See: Naoki Nakaya. "Effect of Psychosocial Factors on Cancer Risk and Survival. *Journal of Epidemiology* 24, no. 1 (2014): 1–6; and S. Tross et al. "Psychological Symptoms and Disease-

Free and Overall Survival in Women with Stage II Breast Cancer." Cancer and Leukemia Group B. *Journal of the National Cancer Institute* 88, no. 10 (1996): 661–67.

"In one oft-quoted study published in the *New England Journal of Medicine* in 1996, a group of doctors watched all the episodes from three popular medical television shows (*ER Chicago Hope, and Rescue 911*) broadcast during 1994–95." See: Susan J. Diem et al. "Cardiopulmonary Resuscitation on Television: Miracles and Misinformation." *New England Journal of Medicine* 24, no. 334 (1996): 1578–82.

"Two recent studies led by critical-care doctors and published in the journals *Critical Care* and the *New England Journal of Medicine* in 2009 and 2010, respectively . . ." See: Hideo Yasunaga et al. "Collaborative Effects of Bystander-Initiated Cardiopulmonary Resuscitation and Prehospital Advanced Cardiac Life Support by Physicians on Survival of Out-of-Hospital Cardiac Arrest: A Nationwide Population-Based Observational Study." *Critical Care* 14, no. 6 (2010): 199; and William J. Ehlenbach et al. "Epidemiologic

Study of In-Hospital Cardiopulmonary Resuscitation in the Elderly." *New England Journal of Medicine* 361 (2009): 22–31.

"**In one study published in 2009 in the journal *Supportive Care in Cancer*, sixty-one patients with terminal advanced cancer (patients just like Helen) and who had cardiac arrest underwent resuscitation.**" See: Christoph H. R. Wiese et al. "Prehospital Emergency Treatment of Palliative Care Patients with Cardiac Arrest: A Retrospective Investigation." *Supportive Care in Cancer* 18, no. 10 (2010): 1287–92. Also see: Elmer D. Abbo et al. "Cardiopulmonary Resuscitation Outcomes in Hospitalized Community-Dwelling Individuals and Nursing Home Residents Based on Activities of Daily Living." *Journal of the American Geriatrics Society* 61, no. 1 (2013): 34–39.

"**A 2007 study conducted by researchers at the National Hospice and Palliative Care Organization and published in the *Journal of Pain and Symptom Management* looked at the difference in survival periods in two groups of terminally ill Medicare patients — those who used hospice** services and those who did not." See: Stephen R. Connor et al. "Comparing Hospice and Nonhospice Patient Survival Among Patients Who Die Within a Three-Year Window." *Journal of Pain and Symptom Management* 33, no. 3 (2007): 238–46.

"Similar results were seen in a landmark 2010 study conducted by oncologists at the Massachusetts General Hospital in Boston and published in the *New England Journal of Medicine*." See: Jennifer S. Temel et al. "Early Palliative Care for Patients with Metastatic Non-Small-Cell Lung Cancer." *New England Journal of Medicine* 368, no. 8 (2010): 733–42.

"Based on these studies, innovative new models of hospice care are being developed in which comfort care is being delivered simultaneously with standard medical care." Most hospice providers require a six-month prognosis for patients with a serious illness to enroll in hospice. This is unfortunate, since patients are left with a terrible choice of pursuing disease-modifying treatments or the supportive benefits of hospice. Two innovators changing this outdated thinking of hospice include Hawaii Medical Service Association (an affiliate of Blue Cross Blue Shield) with its Supportive Care benefit and Aetna with its Concurrent Care benefit. See: http://www.kokuamau.org/whats-new/news/projects; and Claire M. Spettell et al. "A Comprehensive Case Management Program to Improve Palliative Care." *Journal of Palliative Medicine* 12, no. 9 (2009): 827–32.

"During each visit, the patient is hooked with a needle to a dialysis machine through a surgically placed access site on the patient's arm called a fistula." There are predominantly two types of dialysis: hemodialysis and peritoneal dialysis. Hemodialysis is dialysis using blood. The other type of dialysis, peritoneal dialysis, uses the abdominal cavity (peritoneum) to extract waste products by filling the cavity with fluid and then removing the fluid. Peritoneal dialysis is vastly underutilized in the United States as compared to Europe and other places. The reasons for this are varied. Peritoneal dialysis may be a viable option for some elderly patients. For more on the uses of peritoneal dialysis in the elderly, see: Ana E. Taveras et al. "Peritoneal Dialysis in Patients 75 Years of Age and Older: A 22-Year Experience." *Advanced Peritoneal Dialysis* 28, no. 3 (2012): 84–88.

"Close to four hundred thousand Americans receive dialysis and lead normal lives." See: http://www.kidneyfund.org/about-us/assets/pdfs/akf-kidneydisease statistics-2012.pdf. Accessed June 14, 2014.

"And although for thousands of people being on dialysis results in a positive overall experience, there is increasing evidence indicating that many frail elderly nursing home residents with multiple medical issues often do poorly after starting the treatment." The leader in this field is my friend Alvin H. "Woody" Moss, who has devoted his life to better informing all patients about their options in advanced kidney disease. Dr. Moss led the team of physicians and researchers who published the definitive guidelines on this subject used by doctors across the country. For a review of the evidence, please see: *Shared Decision-Making in the Appropriate Initiation of and Withdrawal from Dialysis,* 2nd ed. Rockville, Md.: Renal Physicians Association, 2010; Alvin H. Moss. "Revised Dialysis Clinical Practice Guideline Promotes More Informed Decision-Making." RPA/ASN Position Statement. *Clinical Journal of the American Society of Nephrology* 5, no. 12 (2010): 2380–83; and Alvin H. Moss. "Ethical Principles and Processes Guiding Dialysis Decision-Making." *Clinical Journal of the American Society of Nephrology* 6, no. 9 (2011): 2313–17. I am thankful to Drs. Anne O'Hare, Jane Schell, Nwamaka Eneanya, Michael Germain, and Manju Tamura.

"In one large study published in 2009 in the *New England Journal of Medicine*, nephrologists studied more than three thousand nursing home residents who were followed for twelve months after starting dialysis." See: Manjula Kurella Tamura et al. "Functional Status of Elderly Adults Before and After Initiation of Dialysis." *New England Journal of Medicine* 361 (2009): 1539–47.

"How long would he live?" For more on Art Buchwald's story, read his book *Too Soon to Say Goodbye* (Random House, 2006), written after his kidneys recovered.

"But she acceded to her father's wishes, and we settled on a trial of dialysis to see how things would go." When patients (and/or families) agree to a trial of a medical intervention, it is often referred to as a "time-limited trial," the idea being that a medical intervention will be attempted for a limited time and then decisions regarding continuing the intervention will be made once the risks and benefits of the intervention are assessed at a future time. Time-limited trials are common in the ICU, where, in so many cases, families are the decision-makers for incapacitated patients and feel obligated to attempt life-prolonging interventions.

Chapter 5

"Tom was little different from most seriously ill patients." See: Nancy L. Keating et al. "Physician Factors Associated with Discussions About End-of-Life Care." *Cancer* 116, no. 4 (2010): 998–1006. doi: 10.1002/cncr.24761.

"Based on patients' and physicians' suggestions, these three choices became: Life-Prolonging Care, Limited Medical Care, and Comfort Care." These three categories of medical care (Life-Prolonging Care, Limited Medical Care, and Comfort Care) parallel the work of Dr. Muriel Gillick. Muriel is a world-renowned geriatrician who has dedicated her career to formulating and prioritizing patients' goals of care with medical interventions. Her major contribution to the practice of medicine is aligning medical interventions with whether or not they serve a patient's desired goals. See: Muriel R. Gillick. *Choosing Medical Care in Old Age: What Kind, How Much, When to Stop.* (Cambridge: Harvard University Press, 1994).

"We wanted to create a video that would empower patients and be beyond reproach from medical colleagues, ethicists, and, of course, patients." Ensuring that visual portrayals of medical concepts remain impartial is critically important to the integrity of educating patients. Any hint that the video was nudging people toward one way or the other would discredit the entire enterprise. Thus, a good deal of time is spent adhering to strict criteria regarding filmmaking and how the videos are created. Many of these criteria are derived from t he documentary film tradition. For more, see: Angelo E. Volandes et al. "Audio-Video Decision Support for Patients: The Documentary Genre as a Basis for Decision Aids." *Health Expectations* 16, no. 3 (2013): 80–8; Angelo E. Volandes and

Areej El-Jawahri. "Improving Decision-Making for Patients and F? with Video Decision Aids." In *Cardiopᵤ. monary Resuscitation: Procedures and Challenges.* Leonard J. Doyle and Richard A. Saltsman, eds. (Hauppauge: Nova Science Publishers, 2012); and Muriel R. Gillick and Angelo E. Volandes. "The Psychology of Using and Creating Video Decision Aids for Advance Care Planning." In *Psychology of Decision Making in Medicine and Health Care.* Thomas E. Lynch, ed. (Hauppauge: Nova Science Publishers, 2007). For more on avoiding bias in videos, see: Jonathan Rauch. "How Not to Die," *The Atlantic,* April 24, 2013. http://www.theatlantic.com/magazine/archive/2013/05/how-not-to-die/309277. Accessed June 14, 2014.

"First we deleted all patient testimonials." Despite the fact that most people learn through storytelling and narrative, there is a robust debate in the decision-making literature about the use of testimonials in decision support tools to assist patients in decision-making. See: Anna Winterbottom et al. "Does Narrative Information Bias Individual's Decision Making? A Systematic Review." *Social Science and Medicine* 67 (2008): 2079–88. I thank my colleague Dan Matlock for the many hours we have spent deliberating about the importance of narratives in helping patients make decisions that are concordant with their wishes.

"In order to determine whether or not the video helped patients with a serious illness make decisions that they were comfortable with, some oncologists and I decided to recruit fifty patients with advanced brain cancer into a randomized controlled trial." See: A. El-Jawahri, et al. "Use of Video to Facilitate End-of-Life Discussions with Patients with Cancer: A Randomized Controlled Trial." *Journal of Clinical Oncology* 28, no. 2 (2010): 305–10. doi: 10.1200/JCO.2009.24.7502. Epub 2009 Nov. 30. Erratum in *Journal of Clinical Oncology* 28, no. 8 (2010): 1438.

"Our research team's next study recruited one hundred fifty patients with all different types of advanced cancer . . ." See: Angelo E. Volandes et al. "Randomized Controlled Trial of a Video Decision Support Tool for Cardiopulmonary Resuscitation Decision Making in Advanced Cancer." *Journal of Clinical Oncology* 31, no. 3 (2013): 380–86. doi: 10.1200/JCO.2012.43.9570. Epub

2012 Dec. 10.

"My research group has replicated these findings in numerous studies over the past few years . . ." Over the past ten years, I have spent the majority of my professional career not only creating videos to better inform patients and their families, but also conducting research studies to examine the role of videos in supplementing patient-doctor discussions regarding medical decision-making. The Video Images of Disease for Ethical Outcomes (VIDEO) Consortium consists of many clinicians, researchers, patients, and video artists from medical centers around the country. Our consortium has published a series of studies that detail the effects of reinforcing patient-doctor discussions using videos. These studies have examined the role of video use in a variety of clinical settings (e.g., outpatient, inpatient, nursing home, et cetera) as well as in a variety of health states (e.g., cancer, Alzheimer's disease, heart failure, et cetera). Findings from these studies include the following:

1. Patients who use educational videos to supplement their decision-making about end-of-life care have more knowledge about their deci-

sions as compared to patients who do not use videos.

2. Patients with a serious illness who have more knowledge about their decisions after viewing educational videos often prefer more comfort-oriented medical care at the end of life.

3. Patients who view educational videos about medical care are more likely to have The Conversation with their doctor, and are more likely to avoid having unwanted medical care at the end of life.

4. Patients are overwhelmingly comfortable watching videos and would strongly recommend educational videos to others who are making decisions about their goals of care.

Below, I have highlighted the major studies into their relevant categories for quick reference, along with a short summary of the study. A detailed citation for each article is listed at the end. For the latest publications, please visit our nonprofit foundation's Web site (http://www.acpdecisions.org/evidence-publications/). I am thankful to the many organizations that have funded this work, including: the National Institutes of Health, the Agency for Healthcare Research and Quality, the Alzheimer's Association, and the Informed Medical Decisions Foundation (http://www.informedmedicaldecisions.org). The content of the research and publications is solely the responsibility of my research group and does not necessarily represent the official views of any of the funding agencies.

CPR (Think Taras and Lillian)

"Randomized Controlled Trial of a Video Decision Support Tool for Cardiopulmonary Resuscitation Decision Making in Advanced Cancer." *Journal of Clinical Oncology.* VIDEO Consortium.

This randomized controlled trial studied the effect of the video on one hundred fifty patients with advanced cancer who were visiting their oncologist. Half of the patients were assigned to make decisions about CPR after viewing an educational video; the other half were asked to make decisions about CPR without the video and using a standardized verbal description of CPR. Patients assigned the video were less likely to wish to have CPR attempted compared with patients who did not use the video. Patients who viewed the video also had more accurate knowledge about CPR. Patients were overwhelmingly comfortable watching the video and would strongly recommend the video to other patients making similar decisions.

Advanced Cancer (Think Professor Helen Thompson and Tom Callahan)

"Use of Video to Facilitate End-of-Life Discussions with Patients with Cancer: A Randomized Controlled Trial." *Journal of Clinical Oncology.* VIDEO Consortium.

This randomized controlled trial evaluated an innovative approach to addressing overall preferences for the goals of care among seriously ill patients with advanced brain cancer. Half of the patients made decisions about their goals of care after viewing an educational video, while the other half made decisions after listening to a standardized description of their options and without using the video. All patients could choose among the three general approaches to medical care: Life-Prolonging Care, Limited Medical Care, and Comfort Care. Among the patients who did not watch the video, 26 percent chose Life-Prolonging Care, 52 percent opted for Limited Medical Care, and 22 percent decided on Comfort Care. Among the patients that viewed the video, 0 percent chose Life-Prolonging Care, 8 percent chose Limited Medical Care, and 92 percent chose Comfort Care. Patients were overwhelmingly comfortable watching the video, and every single patient would recommend the video to their friends and family if they had a serious illness.

Alzheimer's Disease (Think Nonna Bruno)

"Video Decision Support Tool for Advance Care Planning in Dementia: A Randomized Controlled Trial." *British Medical Journal.* VIDEO Consortium.

This randomized controlled trial studied the effect of an education video about advanced Alzheimer's disease for elderly patients making hypothetical decisions about medical care if they were to develop the disease. The educational video they viewed depicted an elderly patient in an advanced stage of Alzheimer's disease interacting with her daughters. Half of the patients made hypothetical decisions about their medical care after using the video, while the other half made decisions after hearing a verbal description of advanced Alzheimer's disease and without the use of the video. When presented with the possibility of developing advanced Alzheimer's disease, elderly patients were more likely to choose comfort as their primary goal of care after viewing an educational video compared to patients who did not use the video. Moreover, viewing the video improved knowledge of Alzheimer's disease. The vast majority of patients were extremely comfortable using the video and would strongly recommend the video to other elderly patients making similar decisions.

Inpatient Setting (Think Taras, Nonna, Miguel, Helen, Elijah, Tom, and Lillian)

"A Randomized Controlled Trial of a CPR Video Decision Support Tool for Hospitalized Patients." VIDEO Consortium. http://www.acpdecisions.org/evidence-publications. Accessed June 14, 2014.

This randomized controlled trial studied the effect of the video on one hundred fifty patients with serious illness admitted to the inpatient medical service of a hospital. Patients had all different types of advanced illness, including advanced cancer, heart disease, liver disease, and lung disease, among other illnesses. All patients had a prognosis of less than one year. Half of the patients were assigned to make decisions about CPR after viewing an educational video; the other half were asked to make decisions about CPR without the video. Patients assigned the video were less likely to wish to have CPR attempted compared with patients who did not use the video. Patients who viewed the video also had more accurate knowledge about CPR and were more likely to discuss their wishes with their physicians. Patients who watched the video were less likely to have medical interventions performed on them that they did not want as compared to patients who did not view the video. In other words, the patients that viewed the video were less likely to receive unwanted medical care compared to the patients who did not use the video. Patients were overwhelmingly comfortable watching the video and would strongly recommend the video to other patients making similar decisions.

Chronological Listing of VIDEO Consortium Publications

1. The Video Consortium. "Randomized Controlled Trial of a Video Decision Support Tool for Cardiopulmonary Resuscitation Decision Making in Advanced Cancer." *Jour-*

nal of Clinical Oncology 31, no. 3 (January 2013): 380–86. doi: 10.1200/JCO.2012.43.9570. Epub 2012 Dec. 10.

2. ———. "A Randomized Controlled Trial of a Cardiopulmonary Resuscitation Video in Advance Care Planning for Progressive Pancreas and Hepatobiliary Patients." Journal of Palliative Medicine 16, no.6 (June 2013):623–31. doi: 10.1089/ jpm.2012.0524. Epub 2013 Apr. 22.

3. ———. "Augmenting Communication and Decision Making in the Intensive Care Unit with a Cardiopulmonary Resuscitation Video Decision Support Tool: A Temporal Intervention Study." Journal of Palliative Medicine 15, no. 12 (December 2012): 1382–87. doi: 10.1089/ jpm.2012.0215. Epub 2012 Oct. 25.

4. ———. "A Randomized Controlled Trial of a Goals-of-Care Video for Elderly Patients Admitted to Skilled Nursing Facilities." Journal of Palliative Medicine 15, no. 7 (July 2012): 805–11. doi: 10.1089/ jpm.2011.0505. Epub 2012 May 4.

5. ———. "Augmenting Advance Care Planning in Poor Prognosis Cancer with a Video Decision Aid: A Preintervention-Postintervention Study." *Cancer* 118, no. 17 (September 2012): 4331–38. doi: 10.1002/cncr.27423. Epub 2012 Jan. 17.

6. ———. "Audio-Video Decision Support for Patients: The Documentary Genre as a Basis for Decision Aids." *Health Expectations* 16, no. 3 (September 2013): e80–88. doi: 10.1111/j.1369-7625.2011 .00727.x. Epub 2011 Oct. 28.

7. ———. "Assessing End-of-Life Preferences for Advanced Dementia in Rural Patients Using an Educational Video: A Randomized Controlled Trial." *Journal of Palliative Medicine* 14, no. 2 (February 2011): 169–77. doi: 10.1089/jpm.2010 .0299. Epub 2011 Jan. 21.

8. ———. " 'It Helps Me See with My Heart': How Video Informs Patients' Rationale for Decisions About Future Care in Advanced Dementia." *Patient Education and Counseling* 81, no. 2 (November 2010): 229–34. doi: 10.1016/

j.pec.2010.02.004. Epub 2010 Mar. 2.

9. ———. "Use of Video to Facilitate End-of-Life Discussions with Patients with Cancer: A Randomized Controlled Trial." *Journal of Clinical Oncology* 28, no. 2 (January 2010): 305–10. doi: 10.1200/JCO.2009. 24.7502. Epub 2009 Nov. 30. Erratum in *Journal of Clinical Oncology* 28, no. 8 (March 2010): 1438.

10. ———. "Using Video Images to Improve the Accuracy of Surrogate Decision-Making: A Randomized Controlled Trial." *Journal of the American Medical Directors Association* 10, no. 8 (October 2009): 575–80. doi: 10.1016/j.jamda.2009.05 .006. Epub 2009 Sep. 3.

11. ———. "Improving Decision Making at the End of Life with Video Images." *Medical Decision Making* 30, no. 1 (January–February 2010): 29–34. doi: 10.1177/ 0272989X09341587. Epub 2009 Aug. 12.

12. ———. "Video Decision Support Tool for Advance Care Planning in Dementia: Randomised Controlled Trial." *British Medical Journal* 338

(May 2009): b2159. doi: 10.1136/
bmj.b2159.

13. ———. "Health Literacy Not Race
Predicts End-of-Life Care Preferences." *Journal of Palliative Medicine*
11, no.5 (June 2008):754–62. doi:
10.1089/jpm.2007.0224.
14. ———. "Overcoming Educational
Barriers for Advance Care Planning
in Latinos with Video Images." *Journal of Palliative Medicine* 11, no. 5
(June 2008): 700–6. doi: 10.1089/
jpm.2007.0172.
15. ———. "Using Video Images of
Dementia in Advance Care Planning." *Archives of Internal Medicine*
167, no. 8 (April 2007): 828–33.

**"Patients make better-informed deci-
sions using a video because they see
possible procedures and interventions
with their own eyes."** The use of visual
images to better inform people and improve understanding is not unique to the
practice of medicine. An entire field has
developed around the role of multimedia
learning and how visual aids improve
comprehension of complex ideas. One
very approachable text on the subject is
Richard E. Bayer, *Multimedia Learning*

(Cambridge: Cambridge University Press, 2009).

"In 2009, Group Health Cooperative, a network of physicians and clinics for more than half a million patients in Washington State, started a massive effort to change the culture of care by incorporating twelve video decision aids for medical decisions into clinical practice in six areas: orthopedics, cardiology, urology, women's health, breast cancer, and back care." See: David E. Arterburn et al. "Introducing Decision Aids at Group Health Was Linked to Sharply Lower Hip and Knee Surgery Rates and Costs." *Health Affairs (Millwood)* 31, no. 9 (2012): 2094–104.

"Physicians use checklists to remind themselves of the information and best practices at their fingertips." For more on the role on checklists, see: Atul Gawande. *The Checklist Manifesto* (New York: Holt, 2011); Marty Makary. *Unaccountable: What Hospitals Won't Tell You and How Transparency Can Revolutionize Health Care.* (New York: Bloomsbury, 2012); and Peter Pronovost and Eric Vohr. *Safe Patients, Smart Hospitals: How One Doctor's Checklist Can Help Us Change Health Care from the Inside Out,* (New

York: Hudson Street Press, 2011).

"For instance, many intensive care units have checklists to remind physicians of proper sterile techniques for inserting central lines; and most surgical operating rooms use checklists to reinforce accepted safety practices and to foster better communication and teamwork." See: Peter Pronovost et al. "An Intervention to Decrease Catheter-Related Bloodstream Infection in the ICU." *New England Journal of Medicine* 355, no. 26 (2006): 2725–32.

Chapter 6

"Not too long ago patients with melanoma were given the same grim news that I gave Lillian, and yet two recently discovered medicines can now offer these patients a few more months of life." See: Paul B. Chapman et al. "Improved Survival with Vemurafenib in Melanoma with BRAF V600E Mutation." *New England Journal of Medicine* 364, no. 26 (2011): 2507–16. doi: 10.1056/NEJMoa1103782. Epub 2011 June 5.

"The presence of family members during resuscitation is no longer uncom-

mon in hospitals." See: Patricia Jabre et al. "Family Presence During Cardiopulmonary Resuscitation." *New England Journal of Medicine* 368, no. 11 (2013): 1008–18. doi: 10.1056/NEJMoa1203366; Constance J. Doyle et al. "Family Participation During Resuscitation: An Option." *Annals of Emergency Medicine* 16, no. 6 (1987): 673–75; and Patricia Mian et al. "Impact of a Multifaceted Intervention on Nurses' and Physicians' Attitudes and Behaviors Toward Family Presence During Resuscitation." *Critical Care Nurse* 27, no. 1 (2007): 52–61.

Afterword

"To spark these exchanges and to empower people to understand their options, people have the opportunity to review a video with their doctors and nurses." All 1.4 million residents of Hawaii have the opportunity to review the video in conjunction with having The Conversation with their doctor. The video is intended to augment communication between patients and their providers, not to replace that critical interaction. **"The goal of this monumental effort is to change the culture about this issue**

and to have patients 'at the center of, in control of, and responsible for their own well-being.' " See the vision statement of Hawaii Medical Service Association at http://www.hmsa.com/about. Accessed March 10, 2014.

"As I traveled back to Boston from Hawaii, I reviewed a recent medical study that reminded me how far the health care system has to go before patients are at the center and in charge of their medical care." See: http://www.acpdecisions.org/evidence-publications. Accessed June 14, 2014.

"Invasive medical interventions — like CPR, breathing machines, and feeding tubes — performed without a patient's consent must also be considered medical errors."

The principle of informed consent being applied to medical interventions that patients receive at the end of life that they never wished for is slowly percolating within the medical literature. Disregarding patients' wishes at the end of life should be viewed no differently than other medical contexts. See: Angelo E. Volandes et al. "The New Tools: What 21st Century Education Can Teach Us." *Healthcare* 1, no. 3–4 (2013): 79–81; and Theresa A. Allison and Rebecca L. Sudore. "Disregard of Patients' Preferences Is a Medical Error: Comment on 'Failure to Engage Hospitalized Elderly Patients and Their Families in Advance Care Planning.' " *JAMA Internal Medicine* 173, no. 9 (2013): 787. Also see: Institute of Medicine. *To Err Is Human: Building a Safer Health System,* 2000.

"Until that is achieved, I will continue to 'strive in regards to disease two things, to do good or not to do harm.' " See: Hippocrates. *Epidemics I.*

SELECTED BIBLIOGRAPHY
AND FURTHER READING

Medicine is a journey of learning that never ends; from the greenest medical student to the most senior physician, doctors are continually learning. To reinforce this credo, some hospitals insist that all physicians — from students to the most senior doctors — wear short white coats, the kind traditionally given to medical students. The scene of doctors of all ages and sizes wearing short white coats looks peculiar to outsiders, but it remains a powerful reminder to all physicians of the importance of maintaining humility in the presence of so much disease and death. Each patient is a new textbook, a potential learning opportunity, whether at the start of your medical career or toward the tail end.

As each new patient opens new ways of seeing old things, books also mold one's understanding of medicine over time. Many books I've read since medical school have shaped my understanding of the proper role of death in life. I would be remiss if I did not list some of the books that have shaped my thinking from the time I first wore my short white coat.

They are intentionally not in alphabetical order, but rather in the order in which I read them.

Nuland, Sherwin B. *How We Die* (New York: Vintage, 1994).

Selzer, Richard. *Mortal Lessons: Notes on the Art of Surgery* (San Diego: Harcourt Brace, 1996).

————. *Letters to a Young Doctor.* (San Diego: Mariner Books, 1996).

Katz, Jay. *The Silent World of Doctor and Patient* (Baltimore: Johns Hopkins University Press, 1984).

Ariès, Philippe. *Western Attitudes Toward Death: From the Middle Ages to the Present.* Translated by Patricia Ranum. The Johns Hopkins Symposia in Comparative History (Baltimore: Johns Hopkins University Press, 1994).

————. *The Hour of Our Death: The Classic History of Western Attitudes Toward Death over the Last One Thousand Years.* Translated by Helen Weaver (Vintage: New York, 1982).

Kleinman, Arthur. *The Illness Narratives: Suffering, Healing and the Human Condition* (New York: Basic Books, 1989).

Kübler-Ross, Elisabeth. *On Death and Dying* (New York: Charles Scribner's Sons, 1968).

Edson, Margaret. *Wit: A Play* (New York: Faber & Faber, 1999).

Tolstoy, Leo. *The Death of Ivan Ilyich.* Translated by L. Solotaroff (New York: Bantam Classics, 1981).

Sontag, Susan. *Illness As Metaphor.* (New York: Picador, 1999).

Cassell, Eric J. *The Nature of Suffering and the Goals of Medicine* (New York: Oxford University Press, 2004).

Byock, Ira. *Dying Well.* (New York: Riverhead, 1998).

Gillick, Muriel R. *The Denial of Aging: Perpetual Youth, Eternal Life, and Other Dangerous Fantasies* (Cambridge, Mass.: Harvard University Press, 2007).

———. *Choosing Medical Care in Old Age: What Kind, How Much, When to Stop* (Cambridge, Mass.: Harvard University Press, 1994).

Callahan, Daniel. *Setting Limits: Medical Goals in an Aging Society.* (New York: HarperCollins, 1995.)

Annas, George J. *The Rights of Patients: The Basic ACLU Guide to Patient Rights* (New York: New York University Press, 1992).

Schneider, Carl E. *The Practice of Autonomy: Patients, Doctors, and Medical Decisions* (Oxford: Oxford University Press, 1998).

Gaylin, Willard, and Bruce Jennings. *The Perversion of Autonomy: Coercion and Constraints in a Liberal Society* (Washington, D.C.: Georgetown University Press, 2003).

Didion, Joan. *The Year of Magical Thinking* (New York: Vintage, 2007).

Mukherjee, Siddhartha. *The Emperor of All Maladies: A Biography of Cancer* (New York: Scribner, 2010).

INDEX

A

Abernethy, Amy, 260

Accreditation Council for Graduate
Medical Education, 267

advance directives, 229–37. *See also* health
care proxies; living wills

Aeschylus, 27

Aetna, 282

agents. *See* health care proxies

Alzheimer, Alois, 60

Alzheimer's disease
chronic nature of, 59
health proxies for individuals with, 77–79
history of, 60–61
impairment with, 61–62
and video education, 293–94

American Geriatrics Society, 83, 273

American Heart Association, 87

Aristotle, 27

B

Back, Anthony, 261
Boston, 204
brain cancer, 110–13
British Medical Journal, 75
Buchwald, Art, 141
butterfly glioma (glioblastoma multiforme), 110–16, 151–54

C

cancer, brain, 110–13
cancer patients
  and CPR, 122–24
  having conversations with, 35–36
  hospice care for, 128
  research on using video education with, 292
cardiac tamponade, 42
Center to Advance Palliative Care, 232, 245, 259
checklists, physician, 173
children of sick patients. *See* family of patient
civil rights movement, 134
Code Blue, 13–16, 39, 45
colon cancer, 130
comfort care
  as option, 158, 164
  overview, 227
comfort-oriented approach, 158

P

Q

R

Reasons and Persons (Derek Parfit), 274
religious beliefs, 220–21
residents
  communication skills of, 54–55
  training of, 53–54
Respecting Choices program, 262

S

Society of General Internal Medicine, 83,
    273
Socrates, 27
spiritual beliefs, 220–21
spouses of sick patients. *See* family of
    patient
students, medical, 54–55
Sudore, Rebecca, 246–47
Supportive Care in Cancer (journal), 124

T

Teno, Joan, 257–58
terminal illness, 122
Tolle, Susan, 252

U

University of Rochester School of
    Medicine, 51–52

V

video education, 159–75
  effectiveness of, 166–69, 171–72
  and patient-doctor relationships, 171–72
  PREPARE program for, 246–47
  research on, 159–69, 172–74, 289–300
Video Images of Disease for Ethical
      Outcomse (VIDEO) Consortium, 250

W

Whitman, Walt, 132
wills, living. *See* living wills

X

xiphoid process, 43

ABOUT THE AUTHOR

Angelo E. Volandes is a physician and researcher at Harvard Medical School. He is also the founder of Advance Care Planning Decisions, a nonprofit organization devoted to encouraging The Conversation through the use of videos. He and his wife have two children and live outside Boston, Massachusetts. Visit him online at www.AngeloVolandes.com.

The employees of Thorndike Press hope you have enjoyed this Large Print book. All our Thorndike, Wheeler, and Kennebec Large Print titles are designed for easy reading, and all our books are made to last. Other Thorndike Press Large Print books are available at your library, through selected bookstores, or directly from us.

For information about titles, please call:
(800) 223-1244

or visit our Web site at:
http://gale.cengage.com/thorndike

To share your comments, please write:
Publisher
Thorndike Press
10 Water St., Suite 310
Waterville, ME 04901